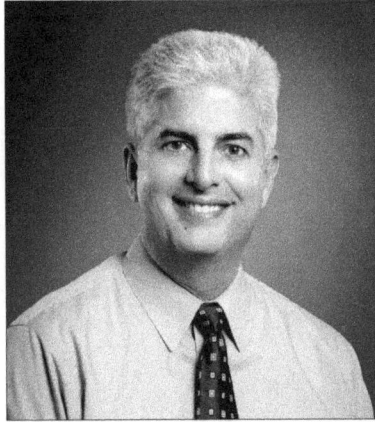

Dr. Julio Gonzalez

The Case for Free Market Healthcare

Dr. Julio Gonzalez is an orthopedic surgeon, former State Representative in the Florida House of Representatives, and attorney.

Born in Miami, Florida, to Cuban refugees, Dr. Gonzalez obtained his medical degree from the University of Miami School of Medicine and his law degree from Stetson University College of Law. He served as a flight surgeon in the United States Navy deploying twice aboard the U.S.S. America to the Mediterranean Sea, the Persian Gulf, Yugoslavia, and Somalia. His prior publications include *Dictionary of Orthopaedic Terminology*, *Health Care Reform: The Truth*, and *The Federalist Pages: A Constitutional Path to Restoring America's Greatness*.

Dr. Gonzalez is married to Dr. Gina Arabitg, a gynecologist, with whom he has two daughters, Monica and Jessica.

Dr. Gonzalez is available for speaking engagements and may be contacted at *gonzopod@gmail.com*.
Learn more at *www.thefederalistpages.com*.

THE CASE
FOR FREE MARKET
HEALTHCARE

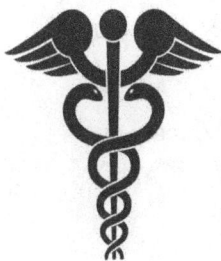

Bardolf & Company

THE CASE FOR FREE MARKET HEALTHCARE

ISBN 978-1-938842-49-8

Published by Bardolf & Company
www.bardolfandcompany.com

Cover design by Shaw Creative
www.shawcreativegroup.com

To

**Gina, Monica,
and Jessica**

Other books

THE FEDERALIST PAGES
A Constitutional Path
to Restoring America's Greatness

HEALTH CARE REFORM: THE TRUTH

DICTIONARY OF
ORTHOPAEDIC TERMINOLOGY

THE CASE
FOR FREE MARKET
HEALTHCARE

Julio Gonzalez, M.D., J.D.

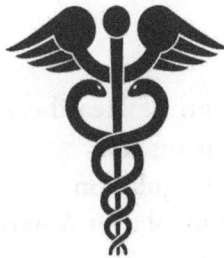

Bardolf & Company
Sarasota, Florida

CONTENTS

Abbreviations

AAMC	Association of American Medical Colleges
ACA	Affordable Care Act; Obamacare
ACO	Accountable care organization
AMA	American Medical Association
ARNP	Advanced registered nurse practitioner
CBO	Congressional Budget Office
CMS	Center for Medicare and Medicaid Services
CDC	Center for Disease Control
CDER	Center for Drug Evaluation and Research of the FDA
CON	Certificate of need
CPT codes	Current Procedural Terminology codes
DPC	Direct primary care
DXA scan	Dual x-ray absorptiometry scan
EHR	Electronic health record (synonymous with EMR)
EMR	Electronic medical record (synonymous with EHR)
EMTALA	Emergency Medical Treatment and Labor Act
EP	Element of Performance
ERISA	Employee Retirement Insurance Security Act
FDA	Food and Drug Administration
GDP	Gross domestic product
GPO	Group purchasing organization
HDHP	High deductible health plan
HHS	Health and Human Services
HIPAA	Health Insurance Portability and Affordability Act
HITECH Act	High Information Technology for Economic and Clinical Health Act
HMO	Health maintenance organization
HSA	Health savings account
ICD codes	International Classification of Diseases codes
IND	Investigational New Drug Application
IPAB	Independent Payment Advisory Board
JCO	The Joint Commission
LCME	Liaison Committee on Medical Education
MACRA	Medicare Access and CHIP Reauthorization Act

MedPAC	Medicare Payment Advisory Board
MLR	Medical loss ratio
MMA	Medicare Modernization Act
NDA	New Drug Application
NHE	National healthcare expenditure
NHS	National Health System (England)
NICE	National Institute for Health and Clinical Experience (England)
OPTN	Organ Procurement and Transplantation Network
PA	Physician assistant
PCIP	Pre-existing Condition Insurance Plan
PRO	Peer review organization
QIO	Quality improvement organization
RAC	Recovery audit contractors
RVU	Relative Value Units
SecHHS	Secretary of Health and Human Services
SGR	Sustainable growth rate
TMR	Transmyocardial revascularization

List of Illustrations

Preface

I first became interested in healthcare policy in 2008. Before that, I was undividedly immersed in the practice of medicine. In fact, my definition of a great vacation read was the latest edition of the *Journal of Bone and Joint Surgery* and the *Journal of the American Academy of Orthopaedic Surgeons*. At that time, political involvement meant meeting my colleagues at my hospital's cafeteria and discussing the seemingly endless interference by third-party payers in medical decision-making. It seemed like no matter what we did, there was an army of untrained pencil pushers waiting to block our recommendations and impede our patients' care. Here we were, whole groups of people who had given up over a decade of our lives obtaining the best preparation possible to take care of those who were sick or injured, and our recommendations were stymied by people with barely a high school education and located on the other side of the globe!

And then there were the lawsuits. Like the rest of my colleagues, I cringed when hearing of the unsubstantiated nature of a medical malpractice action that had somehow made its way to trial. I fomented over the absurdity of medical malpractice laws that would all-too-frequently allow defendants to unnecessarily pay over $140,000 just to say, "See, I told you so."

Also during that time, I served as Delegate to the Florida Medical Association's House of Delegates and Councilor to the American Academy of Orthopaedic Surgeons' Board of Councilors, but those were corollary interests. Yes, those activities were the product of the same angst affecting all physicians over the future of the medical profession, and more importantly, over doctors' abilities to care for patients, but they were activities centered on an interest I viewed simply as extracurricular.

That changed when I read "Call to Action Health Care Reform 2009," a white paper put together by the then Chair of the United States Senate Finance Committee, former Senator Max Baucus. That report, published on November 12, 2008, detailed the Democrats' plans to reform America's healthcare system. It described a scheme so appalling that it demonstrated the immensity of the threat government posed to patients and to the practice of medicine.

Even though I recognized there was something truly sinister about the Baucus Plan, I had not yet gone to law school and therefore not fully understood how it threatened, not just the sanctity of the patient-physician relationship, but also the liberties of America's citizens and even the nation's very fabric. I was also unaware of the full measure of defenses and alternative solutions available to stop these proponents. All I knew was that, as a physician, these solutions were offensive, and as an amateur political observer, I recognized the Plan stood a really good chance of becoming a legislative reality in 2009.

Even more disconcerting, physicians were buying it!

The American Medical Association (AMA), salivating over the possibility of a permanent correction to a flawed physician reimbursement formula, was willing to sell its members' souls for money. It was as if the whole world was cheering an unclothed and villainous emperor as he paraded down the street, and no one, not even those whose very purpose it was to call him out, would!

14

With great urgency, I set out to fight this situation. I began by preparing a set of bullet points for my congressman on how to counter the ideas outlined in the Baucus Plan. Those bullet points eventually became a book, *Healthcare Reform: The Truth*, which I used to attack the Democrats' proposals for reform. *HRT's* publication, in turn, led to a whirlwind tour where I presented the case against centralized healthcare to the public.

But I entered the battle without sufficient knowledge of constitutional or agency law, and on December 24, 2009, Obamacare was passed. The medical world stopped that day as those still possessing any degree of objectivity regarding healthcare gasped at what Congress had just done.

For me, Obamacare's passage posed a difficult decision. I could either go back to practicing medicine and accept the results of whatever political currents flowed before me, or I could continue to fight against the assault on healthcare. I recognized the latter route required my attending law school to obtain the necessary understanding of government, our legal corpus, and the Constitution.

I chose the former.

That decision stood unchallenged for about twenty minutes. My wife, Dr. Gina Arabitg, quickly corrected me and off to Stetson University College of Law I went while running my practice, recertifying as an orthopedic surgeon, serving as my hospital's Chief of Staff, and running for State Representative.

Serving in the state legislature made the power the federal government has over the states even more apparent. There was no way, I learned, to enact foundational reforms for healthcare without running into federally enacted restrictions. The only way to truly address the problems in our nation's healthcare system was to do it in Congress. So, in 2016, when I had the opportunity to run for my congressional seat, I zealously took it, and with that decision, my foray into public service came to an abrupt close. But that loss, although bruising, does not excuse the discontinuation of the defense of healthcare. The forces seeking to control our liberties through healthcare regulation care very little whether any one of us is state representative, congressman, or Health and Human Services Secretary (SecHHS). They only care to place themselves in positions of effectuating the greatest power grab in American history and to do so as quickly and effectively as possible. Only now, their efforts are bolstered by a message of class warfare, racial divisiveness, and social injustice.

Make no mistake, in the battle for the heart of healthcare is entrenched every foundational principle giving rise to this nation. How we define the limitations of government with regard to our health will set the limits on how far we allow government to direct and control our affairs. Indeed, in misguidedly seeking our government's protection for our health's sake, it is easy to cast away practically every civil liberty imaginable. This is the reason the Left pursues this facet of governance so vehemently.

In writing this book, I set out to bring attention to the concerted and coordinated attack upon our liberties and our healthcare by those wishing only to attain greater degrees of power over America's citizens. I aim to demonstrate the destructive effects of government's interference upon healthcare delivery and upon the tenuous relationship between man and government. I close by providing a series of steps through which we may preserve our healthcare delivery system while at the same time uphold those principles that imparted upon the nation its greatness and enshrined upon its people their freedoms.

I am eternally indebted to my wife, Dr. Gina Arabitg, for the guidance, wisdom, and love she has consistently and unconditionally given me in this effort. Thank you also to Jessica and Monica, my inspiration for everything I do. I am also indebted to Rod Thomson for his encouragement and to Dr. Michael Patete for his relentless support.

Also, this manuscript could not have navigated the path from my computer to your hands without the meticulous and patient efforts of Chris Angermann, for whose assistance I am immensely grateful.

And finally, I thank you, the reader, for considering these thoughts. Upon you rests the future of an embattled nation.

Julio Gonzalez, M.D., J.D.
February 1, 2020

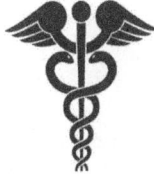

Julio Gonzalez

Introduction

The United States of America stands as the greatest nation in human history. Its greatness is due to the diverse groups of people that would have never attempted to peacefully coexist were it not for an accommodating system of government respectful of their differences. This deference is memorialized in a series of laws honoring their rights and allowing them to freely pursue their passions and realize their dreams.

As we will see, only a free market healthcare system can fit within this system of government, as it is the only one placing the rights and preferences of the individual above all others. Indeed, every healthcare delivery system that is not free market based allows for the priorities of extraneous parties to supersede those of the patient.

In socialized medicine, the priorities lie with the state. Yes, the physician still meets with the patient and identifies the treatments prescribed by science, but the solutions available to the patient are controlled by the government using a formula created by it and influenced by such extraneous factors as the overall value of the treatment to society, the costs of such solutions to the state, political considerations, and most oppressively, the value to the state of the individual being treated. The full force of the executive then enforces these decisions.

In some ways, a corporate-based system of healthcare delivery is even more threatening than one run by the government. Here, the system's top priority is the wellbeing of the corporate entity that runs it as defined by its profits. And although the enforcement arm of the state does not generally back a corporate decision on healthcare delivery, it is also not as easily blocked by the disaffected.

A free market healthcare system is totally different from these collectivist schemes. It is one where healthcare goods and services are exchanged subject to agreements made between the supplier (generally the provider) and the consumer (generally the patient). The prices of such exchanges are set free of any regulatory or external pressures, or interventions. In theory, in a free market healthcare system, there are no restrictions on its participants such that anyone could sell a product or service to anyone else, and any other could be free to purchase it.

Of course, due to the nature of healthcare, such an idealized system of pure capitalism would be impossible to sustain. For one, healthcare is an extremely technical industry with dire consequences in cases of malfeasance, ignorance, or negligence. Accordingly, safeguards must be implemented to prevent such occurrences and to ensure that certain quality standards are observed. Accommodations need be made for persons in life or limb-threatening situations and for those with chronically expensive conditions. These are situations where, if the individual were not attended to, the consequences would be dire, or at least fraught with prolonged hardship and suffering. Quite simply, a Judeo-Christian society such as the United States would not allow for such a cold policy of abandonment and reckless disregard for the state of a fellow human being to exist. Herein lies the natural tension between the business of medicine and the immorality of abandonment.

In the pages that follow, we will explore the healthcare challenges confronting us today. We will examine the assumptions necessary for the creation and maintenance of a workable healthcare delivery system that respects the autonomy of the individual. We will review the history of how America's unique system of healthcare delivery materialized. We will identify solutions to the problems that afflict us and propose rational ways of moving forward. And we will do so in ways that maintain the supremacy of the patient-physician relationship and honor, not only the patient's rights, but also those of the providers who sacrifice so much to place themselves in the position to care for him or her.

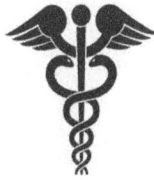

Chapter 1

The Necessary Precepts for a Free Market Healthcare System

Healthcare is hard. It demands that we take into consideration the greatest challenges in life, our most intimate concerns, our greatest sense of empathy, and balance them against those societal fabrics that serve to make a free and just society. Concepts like property rights, religious beliefs, personal wishes, and privacy considerations are entrenched in every legislation made in the name of healthcare.

But healthcare is also an act of charity. In every interaction between patient and caregiver, an individual places him or herself in a position to languish over another. The provider feels his patient's pain. She engages in his suffering and deals with the patient's challenges of confronting illness and injury.

Selfless as the provider's disposition may be, he or she cannot indefinitely engage in this activity without some compensation. There are bills to be paid and innovations to be realized. Loved ones need to be supported and lifelong goals await achievement. If a healthcare delivery system is to be just, it must attend not only to the needs of the sick, but also to the needs of those who toil over them.

A society sufficiently sophisticated to respect and provide for the needs of all involved in the delivery of healthcare must maintain certain immutable presumptions respecting the rights of all individuals. Not surprisingly, these presumptions are similar to those giving rise to a moral and just society.

Indeed, the single most important precept necessary for the creation and promotion of a truly great healthcare system is a fervent belief in God. This belief must include a conviction that this one overarching God is inherently good, that He created man in His image of goodness, wisdom, justice, and love, and that He requires that all men love their neighbors as much as they love themselves. Absent these convictions, there is no second step in fashioning a great healthcare system. Without these beliefs there is no inherent duty to those societal members with whom life is shared. There is no overarching sense of justice. There is no charity. And just as importantly, there is no requirement that human beings reign supreme over government.

The starting point from which a free and just society must be launched is the requisite belief that human beings possess an inherently divine nature that makes them superior to any temporal government. Prescribed governments may rule over the masses, but if man is truly created in the likeness of God, then these governments are inherently restricted in their authorities over those they seek to regulate. Under such circumstances, governments may never encroach upon the dignity and inalienable rights of men, nor can they interfere with the divine nature of each individual.

If God does not exist, then man could reign supreme and so could his temporal government. In the absence of God, it is theoretically possible for the purpose of man's existence to be the state. It also becomes possible for any one man or government to decide the value of another. Healthcare becomes an unconstrained creature of the state, enacted to promote the purposes of the state, and not a resource for the support and benefit of the sick and injured.

As a religion, only Christianity upholds these necessary precepts, and it does so by calling men to love God with all their might, and then, with equal import, by demanding that men love their neighbors as they do themselves. In Christianity, there is a fundamental requirement to care for others, just as there exists the open acknowledgment of God's presence in each individual. Under Christianity, two truisms must exist. First, no manmade entity can rightfully intercede in the interactions between man and God. And second, each and every one of us is organically and individually beholden to the other. Only one economic system may thrive under such circumstances and that system is capitalism.

Yes, capitalism!

You say capitalism is selfish, egoistic, opportunistic and subject to abuses? Maybe, but so is freedom. The very propensities for abuse in capitalism and freedom underscore the great importance of a strong Christian foundation to society. It is this unyielding belief in a strong, benevolent God that tempers man's tendency to engage in abuses against others and turns individual liberties and capitalistic ventures into acts of generosity and altruism.

Sadly, these assumptions, possibly for the first time in our nation's history, are subject to real challenges from those desiring a fundamental transformation. These are the same people who uphold a belief that the abandonment of a belief in the divine nature is necessary to maintaining a free and just society. However, the adoption of natural law is so pivotal to man's free existence that he cannot be stripped of them. Devoid of them, society and government may trample upon any citizen without moral consequence or inhibitions. Indeed, without these assumptions a democratic state respectful of the liberties and rights of its members cannot exist.

Also necessary to a just healthcare delivery system is that its product is not a right. First, healthcare is not inherent to the existence of man. Without healthcare man can continue to exist. Second, unlike common goods, healthcare is not something that passively exists for each individual's taking. Healthcare is the result of countless hours of work by an innumerable number of people without whose participation delivery would be impossible. Healthcare has a finite reach, and as such is excludible and subject to rivalry in possession. Such qualities can never exist in something considered one's own as a matter of right. The fact is that healthcare is a commodity like any other. It belongs to a person or a group of persons who have developed it, labored over it, and readied it for distribution. Their participation in its delivery within a free society must be voluntary, not compelled. It must be lured by the promise of a just reward for the deliverer's efforts.

We are fortunate in the United States that these precepts are central to the nation's founding and to the creation of its constitutional form of government. This brings us to another indispensable premise; the supremacy of the Constitution. Because the American people adopted the Constitution before all other laws, it is the supreme embodiment of their will regarding the scope of powers they are willing to peacefully yield to government. Legally, the Constitution surpasses all other laws and provides a framework for government.

More than any other document, a nation's Constitution defines its nature. All governmental laws, actions, and judgments must comply with the legally adopted Constitution. If one were to discard the Constitution there would be no restrictions upon the intrusiveness and oppressiveness of government and so the free and just society its founders so fervently sought would quickly disappear, replaced by either anarchy or uncheckable oppression.

It therefore follows that if a plan for a given society, whether it is for the physical delivery of goods and services, entertainment, education, defense, or even healthcare fails to comply with the provisions etched upon its constitution, the plan must be abandoned, or the constitution must be changed. In the words of George Washington in his Farewell Address, "If in the opinion of the People, the distribution or modification of the Constitutional powers be in any particular wrong, let it be corrected by an amendment in the way which the Constitution designates. But let there be no change by usurpation; for though this, in one instance, may be the instrument of good, it is the customary weapon by which free governments are destroyed."

In America, any healthcare delivery system must be respectful of the dignity of man. It must respect the property rights of those engaged in its delivery. It must provide the proper motivation for talented men and women with a zeal for helping others to invest the time needed to train in it and remain in it. It must place the patient and her doctor at the center of the decision-making process, and it cannot, under any circumstances, allow external forces to decide who receives and who does not receive treatment.

As previously noted, instituting the provisions that help achieve these goals is supremely difficult, but so was getting to this country in the first place, building it, and preserving it. Achieving and guaranteeing a free, robust, and compassionate healthcare system is just another challenge before a great and exceptional nation. As with any other challenge, it is one the nation possesses the capacity and resources to overcome, but only through strict adherence to the very principles to which it owes its very existence.

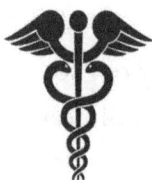

Chapter 2

Healthcare during the Nation's Foundation

From their very inceptions, the colonies had to deal with disease and trauma. The Starving Time afflicting Jamestown during the winter of 1609 is perhaps the first colonial example of devastation from poor nutrition and relentless, punishing violence. The colonist's squalid living conditions led to outbreaks of dysentery and typhoid, among other conditions. The men, harangued by hostile Indians and beleaguered by a shortage of supplies, were decimated such that only 60 colonists out of 300 were still living at the time of the belated arrival of the *Sea Venture* in 1610.

As was the case with self-governance and organization, the colonial experience with disease and its treatment not only readied the new nation for the healthcare delivery challenges that were to come, but it offered the first insights as to what a truly American healthcare system must look like. The concept that no single person ought to be placed in a position to decide the treatment options available to an individual was nearly universally accepted.[i]

---

[i] The Case of Health and Human Services Secretary, Kathleen Sebelius deciding to withhold care from a 12-year-old girl with cystic fibrosis is a glaring exception to this rule. However, as will be discussed in Chapter 5, even here, the court was able to intercede and overrule Ms. Sebelius's will.

Just like the king and his government were not to be trusted with the safeguarding of their liberties, the colonists would have never conceded decisions regarding their health to some centralized authority. Medical treatment decisions were consistently made at the local level, often in consultation with the patient's family. Policy enactments designed to protect the health of the constituents were generally made by the village or municipality. That a colony would look to the king's court or Parliament for guidance on how to handle a public health crisis was unthinkable.

As the nation achieved its independence and expanded, the forms of government changed, but the challenges remained the same. Disease continued to sweep across the nation. Famines and climatological disasters recurrently stressed populations. War decimated many and brought with it its patterns of disease and horrors.

But up until the twentieth century, the nation held firm to the autonomy of actions taken by the various states and localities. Although there were some limited national efforts, the delivery of healthcare and the safeguarding of its networks remained firmly nestled within the hands of the various communities and their governing states, a hallmark, not only of the country's political experience, but of its healthcare efforts as well.

Healthcare in Colonial America

The American colonial experience represents the future nation's first foray in healthcare delivery. At the time, healthcare and medical understanding were rustic at best. As late as the 1770s, there may have been as few as 200 degreed physicians in all the colonies.[1] Colonial physicians were generally trained in European centers such as the universities of Edinburgh, London, Paris, Rheims, Leyden, Vienna, and Halle.[2] Indeed, the North American colonies would have to wait until 1765 before the inception of the first colonial medical school in the Medical Department of the College of Philadelphia.[3]

Largely as a result of their scientific underdevelopment, the colonies' understanding of communicable diseases was underdeveloped, yet communicable diseases were arguably the biggest healthcare menace they routinely faced. Colonialists viewed the plagues and pestilence afflicting them as signs of God's dissatisfaction with them. Consequently, their response was tailored at appeasing Him through fasting, prayer, and humiliation.[4]

In rural areas, the practice of medicine was difficult if not impossible. Physicians had to serve as their own pharmacists. They had to travel, often at great peril, to distant parts, their supplies and medicines housed in saddlebags as they made their rounds.[5] For those that could, payment was made with specie, although this was likely not too frequent an occurrence since actual money was scarce.[6] Physician services were apt to be bartered with wampum, tobacco, corn, wool, pigs, calves, and even colts.[7]

The scarcity of physicians forced people to treat their own ailments. Often, many who were not medically trained were entrusted with the physical and medical care of patients.[8] It was not uncommon, for example, for pastors and ministers to serve as the local medical experts.[9] Midwives assisted in deliveries. Makers of lotions produced and promoted extracts with proclaimed medicinal powers, and colonists looked to the local indigenous population for assistance in combating disease.[10]

And disease would come.

The rampant spread of communicable diseases due to the robust commingling of people from varied and distant backgrounds posed a particular challenge for colonists. Europeans brought with them multiple conditions, some of which had never been encountered by indigenous Americans. Rampant disease and rapid losses to their population consequently ensued with absolutely tragic consequences. The importation of Africans in support of the slave trade provided a conduit for the entry of malaria and yellow fever. In all, the most common illnesses of the colonial period were smallpox, measles, the plague (seventeenth century), typhoid fever, malaria, beriberi, tuberculosis, pneumonia, scurvy, and yellow fever,[11] and the organized response to these illnesses was often scant and ineffective.

Healthcare legislation was reactive, locally driven;[12] and centered on public health measures. For example, quarantine laws were passed in the Massachusetts Bay Colony regarding certain conditions.[13] Nuisance laws such as prohibitions against leaving fish or garbage near bridges or prescribed creeks often had public health benefits at their core,[14] and cities like Boston, Charleston, and New York established quarantine houses.[15]

But no disease had a greater impact on the enactment of colonial legislation and the development of organized preventive medicine efforts than smallpox. Initially, despite clues of an eventual solution to smallpox dating back to 430 B.C.,[16] colonial Americans were largely unaware of the cause of smallpox. By 1630, the practice of taking material from the pustule of an infected individual and placing it below the skin of uninfected individuals with the intent of conferring immunity was brought to the Ottoman Empire by Circassian traders.[17] This technique of "variolation" made its way to London in the early eighteenth century with some success. Later in the eighteenth century, Edward Jenner learned of dairymaids in rural England who claimed that their exposure to cowpox immunized them to smallpox, and on May 14, 1796, he inoculated an eight-year-old boy with cowpox. The boy successfully resisted the smallpox challenge.[18]

Meanwhile, in the British colonies, North American populations were ravaged by outbreaks of smallpox.[19] It would not be until 1701 that Bostonians, suspecting that some diseases including smallpox were transmissible from person to person, enacted quarantine legislation requiring the isolation of potentially infectious ships. They also created sick houses for the isolation of the terrestrial afflicted while providing for personnel to care for them.

The very next year, Boston was ravaged by an outbreak so severe that it killed 302 residents out of a population of 7,000 (a death rate of about 43 per thousand).[20] A subsequent outbreak in 1721 was responsible for 850 deaths out of a population of 11,000 for a death rate of 77 per thousand.[21] Of course, smallpox outbreaks were not limited to Boston or the Massachusetts Bay Colony. The epidemic ravaging Massachusetts in 1702 extended through the St. Lawrence Basin. In Philadelphia, residents wrestled with a major outbreak between 1775 and 1782.[22] And, of course, the effects of the disease on the indigenous population, which unlike the immigrating Europeans had never come across smallpox, were devastating.[23]

Amazingly, it was Cotton Mather, a Puritan minister, who introduced the idea of inoculation to the colonies.[24] Mather apparently learned of the practice from a slave, prompting him to spread the word to colonial physicians. Only one physician, Dr. Zabdiel Boylston, gave the idea any credence. Boylston began inoculating volunteers during the 1721 epidemic. In what may have been the first comparative evaluation between a control and a study population in history, Mather and Boylston compared the mortality rates among patients who had naturally contracted smallpox with those who contracted it through inoculation. They found the mortality rate of the general population infected with smallpox was higher at 14% relative to that of the inoculated population at 2%.[25]

By 1764, Boston was liberally inoculating its citizens such that 5,000 people were inoculated that year. Even the poor were inoculated that year either through the charitable works of local physicians or through the efforts of private benefactors.[26] In New York and Virginia, legislation was passed in 1777 to allow for greater access to inoculation, and Virginia took the extra step of allocating funds for the inoculation of their poverty-stricken population.[27]

Smallpox also played an important role in the Revolutionary War. In particular, a smallpox infestation may have served as a major contributing factor to the failed American attempt at taking Quebec on December 31, 1775.[28] In fact, according to multiple witnesses, the infection of American soldiers likely began on or about December 9, 1775, concurrent with the appearance of infected British spies who may have been sent to interact with American troops for the sole purpose of spreading their infection.[29]

Perhaps in part due to the smallpox epidemic gripping his soldiers, the American Continental Army forces were unable to take Quebec from England. British troops, on the other hand, were left unaffected allowing them to fight much more effectively than the sickly American fighters.

George Washington was made aware of the diseased state of his American troops during the failed Battle of Quebec of 1775. Rumors had spread about the prevalence of smallpox in the American military camps and served as yet another deterrent to signing up for military service.[30] Although at first Washington was anti-inoculation, in January 1777, he finally implemented a program of mandatory troop inoculation.[31] By late 1778, the American military had been rid of the disease,[32] and the young nation's view on vaccinating its troops was forever transformed.

As medical advances took place and the rigors associated with allowing untrained individuals to treat patients recognized, licensure requirements for the practice of medicine and for the participation in the healthcare delivery market were enacted. As early as 1631, Boston punished an individual for engaging in medical quackery,[33] and in 1649, the Massachusetts Bay Colony enacted a medical licensing requirement.[34]

New York followed suit, first in 1760 by regulating the practice of medicine, and then in 1797 by implementing an actual licensure requirement for the practice of medicine.[35] In 1769, Virginia passed a law restricting the administration of inoculations to those licensed to engage in such activities.[36]

Healthcare Developments under The Articles of Confederation

The colonies would declare themselves independent states on July 2, 1776, and on March 1, 1781, would adopt the Articles of Confederation. The purpose of the Articles was to bring together thirteen sovereigns to fight the British and win a war. It was a working agreement governing their interactions and relationships while preserving their independence. As such, the Articles did little to centralize the organizational affairs of the original states. Healthcare matters, of course, remained under the complete jurisdiction of the various states. Even the Northwest Ordinance, the only governing resolution of any significance created by the national government under the Articles, did not make accommodations for the regulation of healthcare of its citizens. Such legislation would have to wait for the ratification of a new document, the Constitution of the United States.

The Constitution and Our Nation's Healthcare

The document that defined America was the United States Constitution. Brought about by the inherent weaknesses of the hastily crafted Articles of Confederation, the Constitution aimed to build a nation. It essentially served three purposes. First, it would be the blueprint of a new government, one that had never been previously conceived. Second, it was to define the limits of the authorities of the federal government. And third, it was to memorialize the protections of certain inalienable rights.

The Constitution's governmental design was meant to inhibit the expansion of power. The Framers developed a system made up of three coequal branches of government. In theory at least, no branch could supersede the other in importance, and each was dependent upon the other for its function. The government was to be layered, such that the national government, with its unifying agenda over the thirteen then-existing states, was only to have certain enumerated powers given to it through the consent of those very thirteen states. These were delineated in Article I of the Constitution dealing with the legislature.

Below the national government, allegiant to it but not subservient, were the states. They were to function as the stalwart of the new system of government. Being that they created the federal government, the states retained all powers and authorities that they did not expressly yield to the new national government. The states remained independent sovereigns and specifically were not departments of the national government. By comparison, cities, counties, and other municipalities were creatures of the state governments, to be created and eliminated by them at their choosing, and given whatever authorities the states felt appropriate. The municipalities were departments of the states.

To the states belonged all issues dealing with the morale, welfare, health, and safety of its constituents; the so-called police powers. Although the federal (national) government was responsible for the common defense, that is the defense of the nation against common enemies foreign or domestic, it specifically was not given the authority to intercede in the inner workings of the states.

Despite there being three physicians in the Constitutional Convention,[ii] the Constitution did not specifically address healthcare. Although one could argue that this was because the field of public health had not yet materialized, the more likely reason is that the Framers had no intention of delegating any regulatory authority regarding healthcare to the federal government. Simply put, in the eyes of the states, the national government was not to regulate the policies enacted by them. The states were independent sovereigns overseeing the affairs of their constituents, and the new federal government was not enacted to intrude on their internal regulatory decisions.

It has been argued that although the words "health," "healthcare," or "health care" do not appear in the United States Constitution, they are indeed referenced in the term "general Welfare," which twice appears in the Constitution. This contention is ill founded. The first reference to "general Welfare" appears in the very opening phrase of the Constitution, its Preamble. The Preamble is an aspirational section of the Constitution, which defends the necessity of its

---

[ii] These were Hugh Williamson of North Carolina, James McClurg of Virginia, and James McHenry of Maryland who is the namesake of the Baltimore fort attacked by the British in the War of 1812 that served as the backdrop for the "Stars Spangled Banner."

passage. In it, the Framers explained that the Constitution was being ordained and established to, among other things, promote the "general Welfare." But in this context, the phrase carries no specific legal significance nor does the Preamble carry any legal authority. It does not grant to the federal government any powers nor has any argument before a court been successfully made underpinning a new grant of authority based on the words in the Preamble.

"General Welfare" next appears in Article I, Section 8, Clause 1, stating, "Congress shall have Power To lay and collect Taxes Duties, Imposts and Excises, to pay the Debts and provide for the common Defence and general Welfare of the United States." This clause lays out Congress's taxing authority. Here, Congress is afforded the power to raise money for several purposes, including providing for the general welfare, but it does not empower the national government to engage in any other activity related to the general welfare. More specifically, Article I, Section 8 does not afford Congress the authority to create or manage a national healthcare system, and it is especially not authorized to create a national reimbursement scheme for healthcare like the one in a single-payer system.

Keen observers may bring up the issue of Medicare and Medicaid as offensive to the restrictions placed upon the federal government. Suffice it to say that although Medicaid is technically supported by the federal government, it is administered by the states. Medicare, on the other hand, stands as a much more direct affront to the Framers' intent, the legality of its existence having never been tested before in the courts.

Those seeking to expand congressional authorities to include the implementation of a mandatory national healthcare system argue such powers are contained within the necessary and proper clause of the Constitution. Article I, Section 8, clause 18 of the Constitution stipulates that Congress is granted the power "To make all Laws which shall be necessary and proper for carrying into Execution the foregoing Powers, and all other Powers vested by this Constitution in the Government of the United States, or any Department or Officer thereof." So squishy is this clause that it has been deemed the "elastic clause" and was the focus of the first major controversy regarding the breadth of congressional authority, a battle pitting no less than Alexander Hamilton against James Madison and Thomas Jefferson. The controversy arose over the federal government's authority to establish a national bank. The expansionist, Alexander Hamilton, contended that the federal government did possess such powers while Jefferson and Madison, the strict constructionists, argued otherwise.[iii]

In the end, Washington sided with Alexander Hamilton and signed the bill establishing the precedent for numerous other federal programs and expenditures not specifically enumerated in the Constitution. Indeed, the twentieth-century Supreme Court would latch on to the results of that debate in its efforts to expand Congress's authorities without changing a single word in the Constitution. Take for instance Congress's authorization of spending in 1936 undertaken with the sole purpose of manipulating the prices of certain commodities. The Constitution does not confer upon Congress such broad authorities like manipulating domestic market prices, but the Supreme Court, in _United States v. Butler_,[37] recognized a wider scope of congressional spending powers, holding that Congress's rights to spend were not limited by the enumerated powers.[38] If the advocates for the creation of a Medicare-for-all model for healthcare delivery hope to implement such a system

---

[iii] I cover this monumental battle in detail in _The Federalist Pages: A Constitutional Path To Restoring America's Greatness_.

they will do so using the expansionist interpretations such as the ones laid out by Hamilton and by Supreme Court cases like *Butler*.

There is another line of legal reasoning through which those desiring the centralization of healthcare delivery may achieve that end, and it is laid out in *National Federation of Independent Businesses v. Sebelius*, the Supreme Court case establishing ACA's constitutionality.[39]

In *NFIB*, the Supreme Court essentially opened at least two doors for the highjacking of America's healthcare, though ultimately it ruled on the constitutionality of only one of these. Article I, Section 8, clause 3, of the Constitution grants Congress the power "[t]o regulate Commerce with foreign Nations, and among the several States, and with the Indian Tribes." This provision was aimed at correcting one of the major weaknesses plaguing the new nation under the Articles of Confederation.

Prior to the Constitution's ratification, the states were free to engage in a virtually unlimited degree of competitive business activities including coining their own money, not accepting each other's currency, taxing imports from other states, and even impeding the passage of vessels and goods from their neighbors. At that time, Congress was powerless to stop these disruptive practices. The Constitution corrected this defect by allowing Congress to normalize trade *between* the states and develop certain standards that would apply evenly throughout the new country so that trade could proceed unimpeded. In *Gibbons v. Ogden*,[40] the first case argued before the Supreme Court regarding the Interstate Commerce Clause, the Court clarified the scope of Congress's interstate regulatory capacity.[iv] John Marshall, the most prolific and influential

---

[iv] Further insight into Congress's regulatory authority regarding interstate commerce may be gleamed from *The Federalist Pages; A Constitutional Path To Restoring America's Greatness* by the author.

Supreme Court justice in the nation's history wrote the Court's opinion and explained that although Congress had the power to regulate business conducted across state lines, it could not regulate those interactions, "which are completely within a particular State, which do not affect other States, and with which it is not necessary to interfere for the purpose of executing some of the general powers of the government."[41] More specifically, he wrote, "The completely internal commerce of a State, then may be considered as reserved for the State itself."[42]

Over the remainder of the nineteenth century and into the twentieth, the jurisprudential posture regarding the limitations of the Interstate Commerce Clause remained fairly static. But the twentieth century brought with it new challenges. The time leading up to World War II was marred by great economic hardship. Collectivist philosophies such as Marxism, fascism, socialism, utilitarianism, and Progressivism arose, and many of those judges inhabiting the nation's appellate courts, including those in the Supreme Court, subscribed to various forms of collectivism.

At the peak of the Great Depression, with the nation's economy in tatters, Franklin Delano Roosevelt, a staunch Progressive, inhabited the White House and, true to form, used government to implement interventions designed to spur the nation's economy and provide jobs to American workers in addition to what was being supplied by the free market. Among these were the creations of the Federal Housing Administration, the Tennessee Valley Authority, the National Recovery Administration, and the Works Project Administration, to name a few, through the enactment of laws such as the Social Security Act, the National Labor Relations Act, the Housing Act, the Food Stamp Act, and the Farm Security Act.

In a move that would set up a historic judicial confrontation over the power of the federal government, in July 1940, the Agricultural Adjustment Act was amended to impose maximum wheat production quotas of 11.1 acres of production and yields of no more than 20.1 bushels per acre upon America's farms. These productivity restrictions were supposed to apply regardless of whether an actor was selling commodities solely within the confines of a single state or not.

One farmer, Roscoe Filburn, who was engaged only in *intrastate* commerce, contested the program as it applied to commercial activities within a state. In his view, Congress was acting outside of its authority by restricting wheat production in his farm, production that he intended to use only within his state. His argument was made stronger in that much of his production was intended for his personal consumption in feeding his livestock.

The controversy went all the way to the Supreme Court in a 1943 case named *Wickard v. Filburn* at a time when the Court's membership had drastically changed to a largely progressive one. In it, the Court laid out a brand new interpretation of the meaning of the Interstate Commerce Clause. In an opinion rendered by Justice Robert H. Jackson (an appointee of Franklin Delano Roosevelt), the Court ruled that Congress's foray into intrastate commerce was appropriate because of the aggregate effect of Mr. Filburn's commercial activity.

Under the Court's new interpretation of the Interstate Commerce Clause, the federal government could meddle with *intrastate* commerce when the regulated activity, in its *aggregate*, would affect *interstate* commerce. To quote Justice Jackson, "But even if appellee's activity be local, and though it may not be regarded as commerce, it may still, whatever its nature, be reached by

Congress if it exerts a substantial economic effect on interstate commerce...."[43]

The effects of the _Wickard_ ruling and its implications upon the breadth of federal power were enormous. _Wickard_ essentially allowed for an unlimited reach by the federal government into the lives of everyday Americans. Taken to its logical conclusion, the federal government could openly and confidently regulate the services its citizens provided, the wages they earned, the conditions under which they worked, the types of products they purchased or produced, the drugs they consumed, and the educations they received; activities that until that point in the nation's history had fallen exclusively under the authority of the states.

It is safe to say that, in light of the Framers' distrust of a strong centralized government, the Constitution would have never been adopted if the delegates had envisioned a federal government with the breadth of powers afforded to it by _Wickard_, but despite that, the Constitution has been interpreted to allow such a top-heavy relationship between the federal government and the states.

From this synopsis, two jurisprudential realities become patently clear. Despite the clear constitutional offensiveness of such expansive congressional powers, legislators and courts have morphed the powers in the Constitution to allow intrusions into state authorities to take place that would have never been conceived by the Framers. Second, in light of the liberties taken in the past by politicians and judges alike, those opposing the heavy hand of the federal government in healthcare cannot readily rely on constitutional arguments to prevent further intrusions. Instead, they must deliver substantive arguments that demonstrate the superiority of a decentralized design for the delivery of care to the citizenry and call out the dangers of choosing otherwise to the people's liberties and their healthcare.

Nineteenth-Century Developments

In the wee hours of the morning of October 17, 1855, in Bloomington, Illinois, a fire broke out in a livery stable.[44, 45] Eventually, the fire consumed nearly a whole city block, and one man, William Green, was killed. In addition, a carpenter named Samuel G. Fleming was injured when a chimney collapsed. Although the details of the event are scant, Fleming sustained bilateral, closed, femoral shaft fractures and was taken to a local pharmacy owned by Dr. Eli K. Crothers for treatment.

Drs. Thomas P. Rogers, Jacob R. Freese, and Crothers were called to the pharmacy to attend to Fleming. The physicians diagnosed the bilateral femoral fractures, and Fleming was moved to his brother's house so that he could be treated.[v] It was there that Dr. Rogers worked on Fleming's left leg while the other two men worked on his right, setting the fractures and applying bandages for stabilization. According to Dr. Reese, he had seen the procedure done by "some of the most celebrated surgeons of the country" and attested that the leg was set and the bandages applied "as was recommended by some of the best authorities on surgery."[46]

After the procedure, Fleming was kept at bed rest, and the doctors visited him daily. He was cared for by his sister, Cynthia Ann Fleming, who arrived on October 20th. She had been instructed on how to move her brother and how to administer morphine for the pain.

Initially, the course of treatment proceeded uneventfully with the patient feeling relatively comfortable. According to Dr. Freese,

---

[v] These injuries predated the development of X-rays, so the physicians would have had to make the diagnoses and direct the treatment of Mr. Fleming's broken thighbones by feel and sight.

"In reply to my inquiries the Plaintiff said he was getting along first-rate, and that, were it not for the confinement, he would scarcely know that his legs were broken-so little pain did he suffer."[47]

Prior to the injury, Mr. Fleming had been suffering from bouts of pleurisy that were causing him chest and rib pain, and he occasionally complain to Dr. Freese about his pleurisy while denying pain to his legs.[vi]

On the sixteenth day, a marked deterioration in the level of pain in the patient's right lower extremity developed. Dr. Edward R. Roe evaluated Fleming, as neither of the physicians who initially attended to him was immediately available. Dr. Roe felt the legs looked satisfactory and treated Fleming with morphine. The next day, Dr. Crothers saw Fleming. He ascribed the deterioration in the patient's pain to worsening pleurisy and not to any particular problem in his legs. Fleming's sister, nonetheless, disagreed. She felt Fleming's right leg had been "misplaced."

Twenty-four days after the injury, Dr. Rogers visited the patient, having returned from a trip out of town. Dr. Rogers' impression was that the legs "were as crooked as ram's horns," noting a three-quarter-inch limb-length discrepancy.[48, 49] Thirty-two days after the injury, when the bandages were once again removed, the right leg was found to be misaligned. According to Dr. Freese, "the right one had a considerable bend at the point of the fracture. The fracture was originally oblique, and now we found the lower sharp point of the upper portion of the thigh bone bending outward from a proper line of the bone when in a sound condition-upon examining, we found considerable adhesions had already taken place."[50] A recommendation was made to reduce the fracture under chloroform anesthesia.

[vi] Pleurisy is an inflammation of the lining of the lungs and can be associated with chest pain.

The next day, the procedure of breaking the adhesions was performed. It did not go smoothly. According to Dr. Freese, Dr. Crothers was in charge of readjusting the limb while Dr. Rogers grabbed the foot to apply the "proper amount of extension." Dr. Freese administered the chloroform assisted by his medical student, Mr. Isaac M. Small. Mr. Fleming's brother and sister were also in the room as the procedure was being performed. Dr. Freese then administered the chloroform until he thought the patient was "sufficiently under its influence."[51] He then cleared Dr. Crothers to begin.

As Crothers began his manipulation, the patient began to holler, begging the doctor to stop. The physicians complied and entered into a conversation about aborting the procedure. During this time, the patient repeatedly pleaded that the procedure not be repeated. The family members present were also disheartened and demanded that the treatment be stopped. Mr. Fleming asked Dr. Freese whether the limb would heal if left alone to which Dr. Freese opined that the leg would likely heal, but would be "crooked."

Mr. Fleming responded that he would rather be left with a crooked leg than suffer any more pain.[52]

Dr. Crothers also explained to Mr. Fleming that if he did not submit to the procedure he would be left crippled and that his leg would be permanently deformed. Despite the warnings and advice to the contrary, both the patient and the family insisted that the procedure be terminated.

The doctors complied, but not before Dr. Crothers informed the patient that by refusing to submit to the procedure he could no longer be held responsible for the outcome of his fracture.

By all accounts Mr. Fleming acknowledged understanding the consequences of his requests and absolved the doctors of any responsibility regarding the outcome, at one point saying that he would only submit to the procedure if a "council of doctors were sent to town," and they ordered the procedure to be performed.[53] The physicians reapplied the bandages and continued to visit Mr. Fleming and care for him. By spring, Samuel Fleming was sufficiently healed to be able to ambulate, but struggled with a severe limp.

On March 28, 1856, Fleming sued Drs. Crothers and Rogers in the McLean Circuit Court for $10,000.00 in damages, initiating case number 1229. Interestingly, Freese and Small were not named in the case, seemingly because they no longer lived in Illinois.[54] In support of his legal action, Samuel Fleming hired a team of six lawyers including Leonard Swett, a local lawyer who was quickly gaining the reputation of being the leading medical-legal practitioner in Central Illinois. Drs. Rogers and Crothers hired the firms of David Brier & Jesse Birch and L. L. Strain and Andrew W. Rodgers. These firms then hired John T. Stuart and a young lawyer named Abraham Lincoln to assist them in their case.

The trial did not begin until the spring of 1857. Swett built his case on the testimony of medical experts eager to besmirch the reputations of their colleagues for their own personal and professional gain. Lincoln relied on research performed by his junior partner, Mr. William H. Herndon, and the coaching of Dr. Crothers.

When the trial started, Lincoln tried to paint the physicians as valiant servants who had mercifully tried to save Mr. Fleming's legs by trying to get them to heal despite the conventional recommendations of the day calling for amputation. During his discussions, Lincoln famously used chicken bones to demonstrate the differences in fracture susceptibility relative to age. As Lincoln broke the pullet's bone, he said, "this bone has all the starch taken out of it-as it is in childhood,"[55, 56, 57] and in another monumental instance, the future president asked Mr. Fleming, if he could walk at all. Fleming answered, "Yes, but my leg is short so I have to limp."

"Well!" Lincoln responded. "What I would advise you to do is get down on your knees and thank your Heavenly Father, and also these two Doctors that you have any legs to stand on at all."[58, 59, 60]

The trial ended in a hung jury and was set for retrial during the next session. The case was ultimately settled and never returned to court.

The Chicken Bone Case was not only interesting in setting Lincoln apart from all other presidents as having been the only one to have defended a medical malpractice case, but it exemplifies many of the problems plaguing medicine during the nineteenth century. Although we see the pharmaceutical advances that had taken place with the availability of morphine and chloroform, we also witness the difficulty in administering deep anesthesia due to the lack of even rudimentary monitoring techniques. Patient care, though aided by the input of trained physicians, was still administered largely at home by family members and loved ones. Technological advancements occurred asymmetrically such that even though some areas in medicine had improved, they were made dangerous due to the lag in technological advancements in other areas. Doctors, for example, recognized the importance of setting a fracture in reasonable alignment, but were unable to optimally assess the results of their manipulations due to the absence of X-ray technology. Even if they could achieve appropriate alignment, they lacked the insight and technical acumen to apply hardware to maintain the alignment. The whole situation coupled with the spread of civil litigation set physicians up for a flurry of lawsuits.

Lawsuits against physicians were virtually unheard of in the eighteenth century. In fact, the first malpractice case ever recorded in the United States was _Cross v. Guthrie_, a case tried before the Supreme Court of Errors of Connecticut in 1794. In this case, a physician was sued for the death of a patient that occurred three hours after a mastectomy.[61, 62] The jury sided against the physician. However, the award of £40 fell far short of the £1000 in damages that were originally sought.

In the three decades that followed, only a handful of medical cases were reported. However, between 1835 and 1865, the legal environment changed radically and a rash of medical malpractice activity materialized spawning what came to be known by modern medical and legal historians as the first American medical malpractice crisis.[63, 64] It must be noted that the term represents a bit of a historical misnomer since the term "medical malpractice" did not come into being until much later.

Multiple factors contributed to the nineteenth-century medical malpractice crisis. First, there was a general disregard towards doctors and professionals based on a perception of the ease with which physicians earned their keep. Over the first half of the nineteenth century, physicians went from being individuals that were held in high regard to being thought of as opportunists who made a living off the misfortune of others. Unfortunately, the public's perception was not totally unfounded.

Poor professional regulatory practices on the part of state authorities allowed many unqualified individuals to practice medicine. Quackery and voodoo medicine abounded. The problem of improperly trained physicians was so commonplace that it led to the retrospective categorization of physicians of the day into "regular" and "irregular" physicians.[65] Regular physicians were those who received their training in conventional medical schools. "Irregular" physicians subscribed to much less tested approaches to the

Julio Gonzalez

treatment of medical conditions. These included Indian doctors, urine doctors, water doctors, steam doctors, and homeopaths. The training for these individuals was quite short and ineffectual, often no longer than three months, yet they would place themselves on equal footing in the community with regular doctors. The ineffectiveness of many of these "healers" and their reputations spawned a general distrust of the American physician that unfortunately enveloped the legitimate physicians of the day.

Reputable members of the medical profession were not absolved from contributing to the crisis. Then as now, some doctors were all too eager to testify against their colleagues, their motivation being the enhancement of their professional standing in the eyes of the community at the expense of that of their colleagues. Like today, these individuals were highly sought by predatory attorneys looking to discredit their physician victims. Additionally, an inadequate medical record allowed many professionals to boast of results that were far superior to the ones being achieved.

Orthopedic cases were particularly subject to legal risk. Contested orthopedic cases were the most common reasons for healthcare-related litigation, accounting for 70 and 90% of medical malpractice cases.[66] Multiple factors made orthopedic cases easy prey for litigation. One was the ease with which the defendant could display the effects of the injury or mistreatment. Additionally, with the recent advent of anesthetic agents, physicians treating musculoskeletal trauma cases were exploring methods of limb salvage as a therapeutic approach for a fractured long bone that had not been previously employed. Oddly enough, it was these superiorly skilled and contemporary physicians that were often the objects of legal actions. Not only was the targeting of the more skilled physician an odd reality of the legal environment of the day, but ironically many of the "irregular" physicians were immune to legal action as there were no textbooks that could be used as standards for their practice.

As is the case today, the threat of litigation brought about advances and detractions in medicine. Medical treatment waivers appeared during this time with the intent of absolving the physician from the legal consequences of adverse outcomes. This was particularly common in orthopedics, where many physicians were advising their colleagues not to treat cases of fractures or dislocations without demanding that the patient first sign a waiver. Also during the nineteenth century, insurance networks materialized to protect physicians from the financial consequences of an unfavorable verdict.

One positive development, licensing requirements were tightened at the state level lending some validity to an applicant's claim of having received medical training. Also, the medical record essentially was born at this time as physicians emphasized the need to document their findings to protect themselves against any future legal actions. Finally, this epoch in America's history also saw the appearance of the AMA, an organization whose purpose it was to promote physician legislative interests and to improve the quality of medical education.

But America had a much bigger crisis at this time. Slavery had finally reached a point where it fractured the nation. Abraham Lincoln, the same attorney who represented a physician in a medical malpractice suit was elected to represent the Union as it reeled from the secession of the southern states.

The Civil War was a horrific experience for the United States with over 600,000 Americans deaths. Once again, the nation's healthcare delivery system was challenged. The chloroform that came in so handily in the treatment of broken bones would prove invaluable in the battlefield, but it was in short supply, and the fast surgeon, the one able to briskly perform an amputation, was still an indispensable commodity for any community and military unit. Incidentally, the field of amputation flourished during the Civil War as physicians learned what techniques worked and which ones did not. Additionally, ambulance systems sprung up throughout the battlefield, and the concept of large hospital wards for the detention and treatment of patients developed.

Still, there were no antibiotics and no antiseptics, and physicians did not understand the concept of microbial infection in the treatment of wounds. Surgical procedures, including abdominal ones, were performed barehanded and in the open air with contaminants and soil, free to traverse into the wound and body cavities. Public health, particularly in the South, was in a deplorable state with dysentery and typhoid caused more casualties than war wounds.

Armed with these experiences, strengths, and shortcomings, the maturing nation set its eyes to the twentieth century. No one could imagine the advancements...and challenges...it was about to encounter.

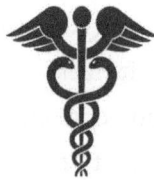

Chapter 3

The 20th and 21st Centuries: The Age of Government Intervention in Healthcare

The twentieth century changed everything.

With its onset there erupted immeasurable changes in technology, culture, religion, social interactions, communications, travel, etc., that would redefine humanity. In the United States, these changes were accompanied by the appearance of the Progressive Movement. An offshoot of the many collectivist philosophies that began appearing in the nineteenth century in response to the pressures of the Industrial Revolution and the political crises gripping Europe, Progressivism centered on the concepts that man's intelligence and the use of reason had sufficiently evolved so that he was now in a position to imagine, design, and implement solutions to the societal problems afflicting him. It was an inherently agnostic philosophy that rejected God and any role He may play in human interaction and the human condition.

If man was able to arrive at solutions for the common good based on reason, then it followed that the most qualified individuals to provide answers were the "experts." Unlike communism whose collectivism was based on class warfare and stratification, socialism whose collectivism centered about the centralized ownership and control of the means of production, or fascism whose collectivism was based on nationalist allegiances, Progressivism was a utilitarian, universal form of collectivism based on the value of reason and pure intellectual analysis. Those with intense knowledge on a topic were the best suited to provide society with the answers to the problems encountered within their field. Although Progressivism appeared to be universally unifying on its surface, it was elitist and did not tolerate non-expert opinions. Thus, if you enjoyed a drink, your preference would be outlawed through prohibition. If you were black, your race would be attacked through a eugenics-based extermination attempt. If you were Catholic, the assault would come from societal pressures and through the repression of your schools at the expense of secular education. Never mind that the weapons used against Catholics would negatively impact Protestantism, Judaism, and other forms of religious worship. While some Progressives would consider such damage collateral, others felt quite comfortable taking down all religions, since after all, the pious were backward and uneducated. They believed in the supernatural, superior beings, and worse yet, Divine Creation.

The traditional societal assumptions that had led to the adoption of certain customs and societal norms were discarded as invalid. Given his intellect, man, by himself, could arrive at the answers to the problems afflicting him. There was no need for gods, overarching commandments (ten or otherwise), ancient traditions, or creeds.

With the displacement of God, there was no need for natural law, no immutable relationship with the Creator, no likeness between God and man, of course, no creation of man in His image. Absent these, there were no unalienable rights because, after all, the concept of unalienable rights bestowed upon man by a superior being would be nonexistent if no superior being actually existed. What rights we had were given to us by the benevolence of the collective under the sage instruction from the experts. And if the collective giveth, the collective can taketh away.

Progressivism with all its supposed virtues was like a ship adrift that while searching for some constancy suddenly discovered it had the most rugged and reliable anchor ever, except that upon deploying it, the ship's sailors discovered that its lanyard was not long enough to reach the bottom. The ship would, therefore, drift indefinitely absent direction or constancy.

Progressivism ushered in the era of agencies and the development of the fourth branch of government. If society needed an answer regarding fiscal economic policy, it would create a panel of economic experts. Our educational system required a team of educators. Of course, environmental maintenance needed all sorts of experts to ensure the quality of the air we breathed, the earth we traversed, and the water we drank. And so government assembled geologists, biologists, chemists, and engineers. And if the problem were social, then a team of sociologists, ethicists, and psychologists would be required, absent any clergy, of course.

Progressivism, with its super-specialized experts, was seemingly tailored to address the challenges relating to healthcare. Medicine was complicated, sophisticated, scientific, and most especially, secular. Experts abounded, not just in numbers, but also in categories. There were experts in every specialty of medicine, public health, and epidemiology, and of course, they had all the answers. So agencies were created to centralize the application of healthcare for the betterment of the collective.

If there was a healthcare problem, then there was a team of experts and an agency that could address it. Thus was born the Department of Health and Human Services, the Center for Medicare and Medicaid Services, the Center for Disease Control, and the Food and Drug Administration, among many others. More than anything else, twentieth-century healthcare policy efforts were characterized by centralization and by the application of the Progressive idea that government needed to control all facets of its delivery, especially its economics.

As we shall see, the effects of centralization efforts are often more detrimental than helpful. In reality, every government intervention is met with some type of tensioned reaction that will either resist the intent of government or bypass it to one extent or another. If government implements mandated price control measures such as price caps, shortages ensue, quality suffers, and/or the black market for that good or service grows. When government imposes regulatory demands without allowing for compensatory adjustments, decreased productivity results. If government places higher quality demands, then low-income consumers get priced out of the market. If government imposes rationing, consumers turn to the black market.

Think of the nation's economy as a living, breathing system. If you stress it, the organism will react. For a biological organism, the stress may be an infection, a wound, or an environmental strain. It's responses, each of which requires extra energy than the organism would expend in an unstressed, steady state. In the case of the nation's economy, every undue regulation, every price control measure or price cap imparts a strain upon its parts. The economy responds by either finding ways of circumventing the regulatory intervention or by delivering the product or service less efficiently. When stressed, the economy must respond with greater expenditures or the target product or service must be negatively altered or abandoned.

The hallmark of the Progressive Movement is that the experts possess the faculties to more intelligently tinker with society's various challenges and successfully chart a way through. But as we shall see, modern experiences with government manipulations of healthcare have often met with predictable negative consequences to the quality, quantity, and price of the regulated product or service.

Medicare

Medicare began with the Progressive notion that government could provide healthcare benefits for all working Americans and their families.[67] Originally proposed on November 19, 1945, by President Harry S. Truman, the original vision eventually morphed into a healthcare plan for seniors.[68] Of course, Medicare was sold as a program where physicians would not be obstructed in the care of their patients,[69] and despite its not remotely fitting within the original framework of the Constitution, Medicare along with Medicaid (designed to assist the nation's poor) ultimately passed in 1965 as part of the Social Security Act.

As originally implemented, Medicare was a two-part program. Part A was an automatic hospital coverage system that would require payroll contributions of about $40.00 per year.[70] Part B, covered physician services through a voluntary $3 per month payment by participants. A concurrently passed third project, Medicaid, was a program of state grants and support that would help them to obtain coverage for low-income families with children, the aged, and the disabled.[71]

Predictably, the program grew. Within ten weeks of implementation, over 19 million seniors had signed up for Part B.[72] But the expansion was not limited to the number of participants. In 1972, Medicare was broadened to include those younger than 65 with long-term disabilities and end-stage renal disease.[73] Home health service coverage was added in 1980 and supplemental insurance created.[74] By 1982, legislation was passed facilitating health maintenance organizations in contracting with Medicare.[75]

Ultimately, Medicare became the largest healthcare payer in the country covering 17.2% of the American population[76] and carrying an annual budget of $627.71 billion.[77]

With Medicare representing the highest number of healthcare consumers in the country, it assumed a position where it could impose an overwhelming influence upon the market. In 1997, it essentially took over the market by establishing a fee schedule and prohibited providers from balance billing Medicare participants.[78] Balance billing is the practice of charging the patient the difference between what the insurer allows the provider to receive and what the physician customarily charges. Although a prohibition on balance billing is designed to protect the consumer, it also takes all negotiating power away from the interacting parties and places it on the third-party payer.

Here's how Medicare's fee for schedule works. First, Medicare generally reimburses 80% of the fee for a covered service, leaving the patient responsible for the 20% remainder. If the fee schedule published by Medicare allows for $200.00 to the provider, Medicare actually pays $160.00 (80% of the fee). The patient is responsible for the other $40.00.

Many Medicare beneficiaries procure insurance to cover the remainder, the so-called secondary insurance, but regardless of whether the patient does this or not, the ultimate responsibility for the remaining 20% of the fee falls upon the patient.

There are services that Medicare won't cover. Many of these are experimental or newer services. For example, in orthopaedics, there is a lot of interest in platelet-rich plasma (PRP) and stem cell injections. Medicare does not cover these because they are considered experimental. As a result, the price the consumer pays for the administration of such injections is directly negotiated with the patient, and the payment comes directly from the patient's pocket.

There is another category of service that Medicare does not cover, but for which Medicare has set the reimbursement fee. The classic situation for this is continuous passive motion machines or CPMs. These CPMs are used after some joint surgeries such as shoulder or knee surgery. In the case of shoulder CPMs, they are essentially chairs with an automated arm attachment that slowly moves the patient's arm back and forth to keep it from getting stiff. Medicare opted not to cover the use of CPMs, but established a reimbursement schedule of the device. Under Medicare rules, providers or suppliers are allowed to lease those for a prescribed amount, but are not allowed to deviate from the price set by Medicare *even though Medicare has opted not to cover it*!

When Medicare prohibited balance billing of its beneficiaries, it set its prices as the end-all of reimbursements. Providers who participate in Medicare are bound by the reimbursement schedules set by Medicare. If the cost of delivering the care to those recipients varies, the provider cannot adjust his or her overhead accordingly, but must eat the costs of any price reductions.

Adding to the complexity of the analysis, Medicare has increased its reimbursement rates at a pace of about 1 to 2% per year.[79] During the same period, overall inflation has averaged

2.16% per year;[80, 81] and healthcare-specific inflation has maintained a 3 to 4% inflation rate.[82] Since physician pay has not kept with either general inflation or healthcare inflation rates, the net effect has been one of continuously decreasing reimbursement such that Medicare now pays about 90% of the costs of providing services to its beneficiaries.[83]

The effects of these interventions have been profound. In those areas where Medicare makes up a small percentage of the market, providers can make up for the shortfall through other sources. In these areas, providers negotiate for higher reimbursement rates from non-Medicare sources, sometimes in excess of 200% of what Medicare pays for the same procedure.[84] This cost-shifting plan has essentially created a silent tax on everyone other than Medicare recipients to fund the otherwise underfunded care of Medicare recipients. In the low Medicare market, the effect of mandated Medicare reimbursement rates on the Medicare patient is higher healthcare prices for everyone else.

In markets such as southwest Florida where Medicare patients make up as much as 70% to 80% of the patient population, the effects of these mandated reimbursement rates are more insidious. Here, the balance-billing prohibition tends to set the market price for services. Since private payers are aware of the Medicare fee schedule and therefore what the regional providers are willing to accept, they will not stray widely away from that schedule when contracting them. Whereas in low Medicare concentration markets, non-Medicare reimbursements may by up to 200% higher than the published Medicare fee schedule, in Medicare laden markets, the private fee schedules do not shift much beyond 105% of Medicare prices. Medicare, and therefore the federal government, essentially dictates healthcare prices in Medicare saturated regions resulting in physician shortages as doctors leave those areas to practice elsewhere.

For Medicaid, the effect is different. Like Medicare, Medicaid does not allow for balanced billing, but with much lower reimbursement rates. As a result, many providers find it impossible to participate in Medicaid programs. For example, in Florida, with the exception of obstetrical services, which are paid at a rate of about 82% of Medicaid,[85] the ratio of Medicaid to Medicare reimbursements span from 48% to 53%.[86] Consequently, only 62.2% of physicians report accepting new Medicaid patients[87] as compared 81.7% for Medicare patients.[88] Thus, low compensation is the reason most physicians do not accept new Medicaid patients (55.4%).[89] This compares to Medicare where a full practice is the reason a plurality of physicians cite for not accepting new patients (37.0%).[90] Also, as noted in Figure 3-1, the percentage of physicians not accepting new Medicaid patients closely correlates with the level of Medicaid reimbursement for that state.

One final consideration is the percentage of providers opting out of Medicare, which has steadily grown from 0.42% of eligible providers between 1998 and 2002 to 4% of physicians in 2016.[91] Based on the data, one can conclude that although physicians are choosing to opt out of Medicare in greater numbers than they did 15 years ago, the Medicare reimbursement-to-cost ratio has not yet to reach a critical level. It is reasonable to expect, however, that if provider reimbursement rates continue to decrease relative to inflation, at some point the critical value will be reached where physicians will start leaving Medicare in high number and Medicare patients' access to care will be threatened.

**Figure 3-1: Correlation between State Standings on
Medicaid Access and Reimbursement.**

Bottom 5 States	% Not Accepting Medicaid Pts	Reimbursement % Range
New Jersey	32.20%	35%-53%
Texas	29.90%	58%-85%
Florida	29.10%	48%-82%
Georgia	23.70%	65%-99%
California	22.10%	41%-76%
Top 5 States	% Not Accepting Medicaid Pts	Reimbursement % Range
Idaho	1.50%	88%-100%
Vermont	2.10%	78%-84%
South Dakota	2.90%	71%-1.11%
Montana	2.90%	1.09%-1.17%
Wyoming	3.20%	98%-1.04%

Sources: "Medicaid to Medicare Fee Index," Kaiser Family Foundation (blog) accessed Jun 15, 2019, http://www. .kff.org/medicaid/state-indicator/medicaid-to-medicare-fee-index/?currentTimeframe=0&sortModel=%7B"colId":"Location","sort":"asc"%7D.; Kelly, Greg, "Medicare and Medicaid Participation Rates for Doctors by State," *MD Magazine*. (blog), Oct. 19, 2016; accessed Jun. 15, 2019, https://www.mdmag.com/physicians-money-digest/columns/the-doctor-report/10-2016/medicare-and-medicaid-participation-rates-for-doctors-by-state.

Another impediment to provider participation in Medicare is the administrative toll of complying with the myriad of Medicare provisions presently in existence. Medicare regulations make up 1,906, two-column pages in the Federal Register. They are continuously updated, published at least yearly, modified by amendment throughout the year, and enforceable by the full might of the federal government. It is impossible to keep up with this continuously shifting regulatory quicksand while practicing medicine, and even if one could, the toll of trying to do so would be overwhelming. For this reason in a statewide poll conducted by the state of Florida, the two administrative subcategories, "Billing Requirements" and "Too Much Paperwork," were the reasons 38.5% of physicians in Florida who did accepting new Medicare patients refused to participate; almost twice as many as those who did so because of reimbursement concerns.[92]

Then there is the issue of Medicare's overt interference with the practice of medicine. The opening section of the Medicare statutes, section 42 U.S.C. §1935, asserts, "Nothing in this subchapter shall be construed to authorize any Federal office or employee to exercise any supervision or control over the practice of medicine or the manner in which medical services are provided, or over the selection, tenure, or compensation of any officer or employee of any institution, agency, or person providing health services; or to exercise any supervision or control over the administration or operation of any such institution, agency, or person." Ostensibly, this broadly worded prohibition would make it illegal for Congress to exert its will upon the manner in which physicians practice medicine.

But this was insufficient to stop Medicare's interference in the name of "quality." From the very beginning, Medicare imposed conditions for participation on hospitals.[93] Later, the implementation of payments based on diagnosis-related groups (DRGs) created incentives for hospitals to cut lengths of stay and move care to the outpatient setting.[94]

To carry out its overseeing authority, Medicare contracted private contractors. These contractors added to their oversight capabilities through quality improvement organizations (QIOs) and peer review organizations (PROs) whose responsibility it was to evaluate everything from readmission rates and discharge data to the "quality of care" delivered by providers. But the work, predictably, was tedious and voluminous, and there were difficulties comparing performance data between providers.

As technology advanced and care measures became easier to track, a more comprehensive method of quality tracking followed. In 2009, Congress passed the High Information Technology for Economic and Clinical Health (HITECH) Act. The HITECH Act essentially pushed for the adoption of electronic medical records and the meaningful use of interoperable electronic health records (EHRs). The goal of the program was to have Medicare participants employ EHR platforms that would allow for the exchange of health information, which, it was thought, would improve health quality and reduce the incidence of medical errors.[95] The program included the creation of grants and incentive payments to providers ranging from $44,000.00 over 5 years to $63,750.00 over 6 years to motivate providers to purchase and install EHR programs in their practices.[96] Although the program was initially voluntary, failure to join by 2015 would result in a 1% pay reduction, and by 2017, those failing to implement EHRs in their institutions would receive a 3% pay reduction.[97]

By this point, the concept of supervising and controlling, or at the very least, influencing the practice of medicine had taken root. As the CDC puts it, "HITECH is a powerful opportunity for public health. With a phased approach, by 2015 public health will have more and stronger partners working to improve population health. There is an increased opportunity to reduce disparities, control chronic diseases, and build a health-promoting healthcare system that is accountable for the health of our communities and our country."[98] A clearer testament of Medicare's self-adopted role of directing the manner in which medicine is practiced in the United States could scarcely be made.

Plenty of other evidence exists demonstrating that Medicare is actively engaged in controlling the practice of medicine. Consider a procedure called transmyocardial revascularization (TMR) where a heart doctor uses a tiny laser to bore tiny holes into a heart's muscle with the aim of restoring blood flow to ischemic regions of a patient's heart. In its discussions regarding the reimbursement for this procedure, the Center for Medicare and Medicaid Services (CMS) wrote, "CMS has concluded that, for patients with severe angina,...for whom all other medical therapies have been tried or evaluated and found insufficient, TMR offers sufficient evidence of its medical effectiveness to treat the symptomatology. The CMS therefore covers TMR as a late or last resort for patients with severe...angina."[99]

This ruling, a routine one for CMS, goes well beyond the relatively passive determination of health quality standards. In the TMR example, as it has on countless other occasions, CMS has reviewed very specific medical data, passed judgment on the meaning of the data, and decided on the indications for the use of that technology. This scientific analysis and judgment are at the core of the process that physicians undergo in practicing medicine. Yet, in this case, that process was undertaken at the bureaucratic level and memorialized in a rule instructing physicians on the circumstances under which their patients may benefit from the procedure.

CMS will argue that it is not prohibiting anything, that it is merely stating the circumstances under which it will pay for a procedure, but functionally, with its balance billing restrictions and the heavy reliance by Medicare beneficiaries on Medicare funding, such a rule effectively places the federal government in the position of determining who is eligible for this treatment and when.

Another example of Medicare inappropriately interfering with the practice of medicine is the Two-Midnight Rule. Whether someone is actually an inpatient at a hospital is pivotal to determining the amount the patient is personally charged for the hospitalization and how the hospital gets paid. This is because, as previously noted, an inpatient hospitalization is covered under Medicare Part A while outpatient services are covered under Medicare Part B. Importantly, only if a patient spends three "inpatient" days in a hospital is he or she eligible for Medicare coverage of his or her post-hospitalization stay at a skilled nursing facility (a nursing home or a rehab center). If the days he or she spends in the hospital do not amount to three "inpatient" days, then the patient is personally responsible for the costs of that post-hospitalization stay, a sum often exceeding $10,000.00.

Therefore, the determination of whether a patient's hospitalization constitutes an inpatient stay is of fundamental importance, and the answer to that question is mired in controversy. For example, if a patient is admitted to the hospital for a 15-minute carpal tunnel release (a minor surgery to the patient's hand) and is sent home a few hours after the admission, such an event would clearly be an outpatient event. Alternatively, if a patient is admitted to the intensive care unit on a ventilator and ends up spending two weeks in the hospital with pneumonia such a hospitalization would clearly be an inpatient admission.

But how about the myriad of other cases in between? How about when a debilitated patient is admitted to the hospital with a broken shoulder that causes her to be unable to go home and has to spend seven days in the hospital? Is this an inpatient stay or an outpatient one? Or how about a frail, elderly woman with early dementia that falls, breaking her pelvis and making her too weak to go home? Every healthcare provider involved in her care knows that after her hospitalization she needs to go to a skilled nursing facility because she cannot be taken care of anywhere other than a hospital or an extended care facility. Should this patient be considered an outpatient even though she spends days in the hospital?

CMS, and, by extension, HHS has struggled with this question. Medicare considers a hospitalization "inpatient" when the condition requires "inpatient services." In other words, when the patient requires treatment that ought only be delivered in a hospital setting. By federal statute, the primary determinant of the need for inpatient services is the attending physician such that when the physician provides an order for the hospital to admit the patient as an "inpatient," then generally, the patient is considered an inpatient. Upon being discharged, the hospital could then bill Medicare for an inpatient hospitalization.

The problem arises because HHS and CMS have authorized Medicare to deny a claim for inpatient services due to the unreasonableness of the inpatient determination.[100] Predictably, this has led to an ongoing argument over whether a particular admission represents an inpatient event versus something else. In 2013, CMS attempted to solve the problem by implementing the Two-Midnight Rule. Under this regulation, any hospitalized patient who the admitting physician reasonably believes will be hospitalized for a period of time crossing two midnights is considered an inpatient for billing purposes. Although the decision regarding the admission status is left to the admitting physician, "[t] he expectation of the physician should be based on such complex medical factors as patient history and comorbidities, the severity of signs and symptoms, current medical needs, and the risk of an adverse event."[101]

But the Medicare regulation instituting the Two-Midnight Rule included an exception. It allowed Medicare to audit admissions to determine whether the status determination, *in Medicare's opinion*, was appropriate. In other words, Medicare could disagree with the physician, and overrule the doctor.

Medicare consequently hired Recovery Audit Contractors, or RACs to enter a participating hospital, review a series of charts and determine the monetary value of the discrepancies they identified in their judgment. That number multiplied by the fraction of the total charts they reviewed was the amount the facility would have to pay Medicare within 30 days to atone for its discrepancies. Adding to the skewed nature of Medicare's review process of hospitals and their billing practices, RAC audits were only performed to investigate inpatient claims and never for claims where an observation or outpatient status was billed.[102]

As one can imagine, an unfavorable RAC audit could be a painful development for any facility, and potentially devastating to a small one.[vii] Consequently, hospitals became increasingly aggressive in classifying their admissions as outpatient or observation statuses because they knew that as long as they erred in the outpatient direction there would be no negative consequences from the RACs. This predictable attitude also had the intended effect of placing a larger burden of the cost of the hospitalization on the patient, and less on Medicare.

To help avoid improper inpatient classifications, many hospitals relied on commercially available screening tools *as directed by Medicare*.[103] Per these billing guides, hospitals began overriding physician determinations of a patient's admission status. Patients who were reasonably believed by their admitting physician to require two midnight stays in the hospital were being denied their inpatient status by the hospitals. Recall, however, that neither

---

[vii] Medicare stopped performing RAC audits on October 1, 2013, only to resume the practice on January 1, 2016, but only in response to cases of persistent noncompliance. Memo of Decision, *Alexander v. Azar*, No. 3:11-cv-1703, (MPS), 12-13 (USDC CN Mar. 27, 2019).

federal statutes nor CMS regulations allow hospitals to override the physician's determination, but they did so anyway to avoid punishment from Medicare through their RACs.

The financial consequences to patients were stark, inclusive of a lack of access to post-hospitalization skilled nursing facility coverage by Medicare,[viii] but its interventions became even more direct when it implemented the "inpatient only" list. CMS created an exception to the Two-Midnight Rule for procedures the Secretary of HHS (SecHHS) deemed to always require inpatient care.[104] For example, if one were to undergo a total hip replacement (THR) it would automatically be considered an inpatient procedure. On the other hand, a total knee replacement (TKR), which is about as taxing on the patient as a hip replacement, is considered an outpatient procedure.

There are several problems, both conceptually and functionally, with the inpatient procedure exemption. First, the rule goes against CMS's prohibition of not interfering with the practice of medicine. If no federal employee is allowed to supervise or control the practice of Medicine under 42 USC §1395, then, by what authority is the SecHHS able to determine which procedures exclusively *require* inpatient services? Clearly, SecHHS cannot make such a determination without performing a supervisory or controlling role over the practice of medicine.

Second, some of the procedures denoted by the SecHHS as belonging to the inpatient-only list are already being performed in an outpatient setting. Hip replacements are routinely performed in some same-day surgery centers for patients covered by private

---

[viii] As of this writing, a class action lawsuit called *Alexander v. Azar* put forth by disaffected patients is being tried in Connecticut's federal district court. The litigation, already eight years old, has no foreseeable end in sight.

insurances even though Medicare lists the procedure as "inpatient only."[105] As a result of its arbitrary determination on THRs, Medicare is keeping its beneficiaries from enjoying the cost savings associated with outpatient surgery centers like private paying patients do.

Similarly, by what authority does Medicare determine that TKR patients ought to be outpatients? If a patient is admitted to the hospital for a knee replacement, the burden falls on the physician to prove to Medicare that the patient requires an "inpatient stay" *ahead of the hospitalization*! If Medicare or its agent (the hospital) disagrees with the physician, then the patient is deemed an outpatient and will bear a higher out-of-pocket burden for his procedure.[106]

Once again, Medicare continues to tip the scales, behind the scenes, to manipulate the practice of medicine in its favor and to shift the cost of care away from its coffers and into those of the patients and their providers. It does this because it has an inherent conflict of interest between the care demands it was created to address, and the taxpayer dollars it is supposed to scrupulously manage. But notice that nowhere in this equation do we encounter the patient's desires or wishes.

Yet none of these actions compare in their obtrusiveness to the creation of the Independent Payment Advisory Board (IPAB) passed by the Democratic Congress under President Obama. For the Democrats in Congress, Medicare expenditures needed to be curtailed and IPAB was their answer of how to accomplish this.

IPAB was to be made up of fifteen individuals appointed by the President, with the advice of the Senate, whose function it was to cut Medicare expenditures when those expenses were predicted to increase more than the rate of per capita economic growth plus

1%. The law prohibited the Board from achieving cuts through rationing of care, raising taxes, cutting benefits, or altering eligibility requirements, but IPAB was allowed to cut provider reimbursements or deny specific treatments on the grounds of cost effectiveness.[107] IPAB was particularly threatening because it placed a group of unelected, unaccountable bureaucrats in the role of deciding what expenditures would be cut. The Board's decisions would not be reversible by any overseeing committee or agency, nor were they subject to the court's jurisdiction. In fact, the only methods of reversing an IPAB decision were through an act of Congress, or a three-fifths vote of the Senate.[108] These brazen provisions were not only laughable, but also indicative of the extent government officials and policy designers were willing to go to intrude into the privacy and rights of Medicare beneficiaries.

The IPAB program brought to fore a number of very disconcerting realities about the Left. First, Progressives were willing to erase Americans' due process rights if it would achieve their cost containment goals. Second, their actions demonstrated their willingness to target senior citizens. Third, they displayed their disposition of hitting providers even if they weren't the cause of a problem. And finally, the deceitfulness of liberalism was displayed, a point exemplified by the passage of a law prohibiting IPAB from rationing care without defining the term so that there no legal description exists of what the Board was prohibited from doing!

Fortunately, IPAB's passage was met with staunch criticisms from those who value human rights and a system of checks and balances. Its repeal would have to wait for President Obama's departure from the White House who stubbornly warned of vetoing any attempt at repealing it. On February 9, 2018, IPAB was repealed before it could be deployed.[109]

Medicaid

To address the care of the indigent and the disabled, Congress created Medicaid. Medicaid is not a pure healthcare system as is Medicare. Rather, it is a support system designed to assist low-income individuals generally. Although the federal government funds approximately 60% of a state's Medicaid program,[110] it is actually administered by the states, which are obligated to comply with many of the federally mandated conditions for participation. Thus, although variations exist between the Medicaid programs in the various states, some general observations can be made.

First, approximately 45% of physicians report accepting new Medicaid patients nationally.[111] Although administrative considerations are a deterrent to provider participation, as opposed to Medicare, the principal reason for poor provider participation in Medicaid programs is inadequate reimbursement.[112, 113] Balance-billing restrictions also add to the difficulty in provider recruitment. As a result, access is a significant issue for beneficiaries. Throughout the nation, Medicaid patients encounter much greater difficulties securing appointments with doctors than non-Medicaid patients.[114, 115]

Some argue that access to care amongst Medicaid patients is better than in the uninsured population,[ix, 116] but this question is still unresolved. Take for example the Oregon Experiment. In 2008, after having closed its Medicaid program for four years, Oregon decided it would reopen its enrollment. From a list of 90,000 people with

---

[ix] The evaluation of healthcare access is very difficult and no definitive answer has been reached regarding the access to care. At least one study reported improved access to healthcare following the Affordable Care Act compared. Veri Seo, Travis P. Baggett, et al. "Access To Care Among Medicaid And Uninsured Patients in Community Health Centers After The Affordable Care Act. *BMC Health Services Research*, vol. 19:291 https://doi.org/10.1186/s12913-019-4124-z 8 May 2019.

incomes of 100% federal poverty level or below, the state random-ly selected 30,000 able-bodied persons between the ages of 19 and 64 who were otherwise uninsured and ineligible for other public in-surance to become new Medicaid enrollees. A study was fashioned monitoring health outcomes of 20,745 people (the 10,405 lottery winners and 10,340 non-winners).

After two years, there were no statistically significant differ-ences between those who were insured under Medicaid and those who had no insurance with regard to cholesterol levels, hyper-tension, glycated hemoglobin levels, the incidence of depression, medication inventories, self-reported diagnoses, health status, healthcare utilization, and out-of-pocket spending on health.[117] What's more, the Medicaid group spent 35% more (or $1,172 per patient per year) than the uninsured group in prescription drug allocations and office visits.[118] So, even though the Medicaid group was associated with more spending, prescriptions, and doc-tor visits, these greater resource allocations resulted in no measur-able differences in health.

Even worse, another study reviewing outcomes from the Na-tional Inpatient Database, Medicaid patients demonstrated a higher mortality rate, postoperative wound infection rates, gastro-intestinal complication rates, infection rates, and systemic compli-cation rates than uninsured patients.[119] Medicaid patients also had higher hospital lengths of stay and total costs of care compared to uninsured patients,[120] making the Medicaid patient worse off than the uninsured patient! Although there could be factors within the Medicaid population pushing towards poorer outcomes, these studies, along with many others, provide only mixed evidence in support of the contention that Medicaid helps improve the health of a state's patient population.

Government Regulation of Healthcare Insurance

Progressives did not limit their efforts at manipulating the markets to the mere creation of government programs. They attacked the private healthcare insurance market as well.

Government's initial interferences with the private healthcare insurance market were the result of a historical accident. During World War II with its colossal dependence on young men to prosecute the war against the Axis Powers, American workers were in high demand. Salaries were increasing, and with them, the threat of runaway inflation. To keep these trends in check, Congress passed the Stabilization Act of 1942 giving the President the authority to freeze wages and salaries.[121] Within a day of its passage, President Roosevelt froze workers' salaries.

Immediately, employers found themselves devising new and innovative ways to attract employees. Many turned to health insurance benefits. Of course, paying for one's health insurance did not equate to a pay raise, but it did provide a benefit for which the employee no longer had to pay. Predictably, the number of insured Americans rose from a mere 9.8% in 1940 to nearly 30% six years later,[122] and by the 1960s, 80% of Americans had some form of health insurance.[123]

As healthcare coverage programs evolved, some companies found it beneficial to self-fund their employees' healthcare. Under this plan, a large employer would administer its own health insurance rather than buy a plan from a third party payer like Blue Cross and Blue Shield, or Humana.

But there were problems. Some employees were dissatisfied that the employer could change their benefits without their consent.[124] In other cases, certain employees would not be eligible for their workplace's healthcare insurance if they suffered from certain conditions, and because the law treated employer-funded health insurance as a gifted benefit, employees had few rights in the face of unilateral decisions. In response, in 1974, Congress passed the Employee Retirement Insurance Security Act (ERISA) as a pension oversight law with provisions pertaining to employer-funded healthcare insurance included in the legislation.[125]

ERISA resulted in a very awkward legislative environment. It left the substance of what was being offered by employer-funded healthcare insurance plans virtually untouched while allowing the states to regulate non-self-funded employer healthcare insurance plans.[126] Predictably, dissatisfaction grew among consumers with the private payer insurance industry. Issues like the spiraling costs of premiums, portability, and the exorbitant price of individual insurance plans dominated the national discussion. Additionally, questions over the best approach of handling coverage for people with pre-existing conditions arose.

With the 1980s and 1990s, the number of uninsured in the United States climbed, and legislators once again turned to the heavy hand of government. In 1996, the federal government passed the Health Insurance Portability and Affordability Act (HIPAA). Again, it left the regulation of private insurance in the hands of the states. But HIPAA did include health information protections and limited the rejection of coverage for pre-existing conditions to a maximum of 12 months following enrollment. But the program failed to stem the tide of the spiraling costs of insurance premiums, and by 2010, the population of uninsured individuals grew to approximately 47 million people.[127]

Seeing this, Congress once again went after the private healthcare insurance market, this time through the passage of the ACA in 2010. The ACA was revolutionary in its scope since it represented the first time the federal government directly regulated private health insurance. The ACA aimed to improve access to healthcare insurance by creating a labyrinthine network of government regulations designed to make healthcare insurance more affordable to the general public. The basic foundation of the ACA was that everyone should have healthcare insurance even if it meant collectively sharing in the responsibility of providing it.[128] If private payers could be artificially supported in funding the nation's healthcare expenses, then the overall strain upon individuals desiring to buy healthcare insurance could be lowered and the uninsured population would decrease. But the philosophy was inherently socialistic, directly leading to further inefficiencies and strains.

Through the ACA created a virtual destination where consumers could purchase healthcare insurance (the healthcare marketplace). The degrees of coverage that the participating plans would offer were divided into four levels: bronze, silver, gold, and platinum. If a consumer failed to purchase one of those four levels of coverage, a penalty would be charged for noncompliance. Private payers (insurance companies) would be allowed to continue to exist, but plans not meeting governmental specifications would not qualify for tax deductions, thus pressuring private payers into providing the coverage the government mandated. The prices insurers were allowed to charge for the various qualifying products were also regulated.

In exchange for agreeing to the pricing and plan restrictions, the government subsidized insurance companies with the revenues collected from those persons and entities failing to obtain qualified healthcare. Additionally, to keep insurance from being inaccessible to higher-risk consumers, "underwriting," or the process by which insurance companies adjust premiums based on a patient's pre-existing conditions, would be eliminated.

The ACA essentially created two categories of individual health-care insurance participants: 1) those who were likely to be health-care consumers such as the aged; and 2) those who were unlikely to be healthcare consumers like the young and athletic. For those who were likely to be healthcare consumers, their choice was straight-forward. They would purchase insurance just like they did before the passage of the ACA, but their coverage options were limited to those defined in the government's four plans.

Those who were unlikely to consume healthcare could either purchase healthcare insurance (even though they may not have otherwise purchased it), or they could opt to not purchase insurance and pay a penalty instead. Whether by penalty or by moneys paid directly to the insurer, the young and healthy would now be paying money without a foreseeable benefit. Upon them fell the burden of "spread[ing] the wealth" about which then-candidate Obama spoke to Joe the Plumber.[129]

The ACA also captured employers within its mandates. Any business employing 50 or more full-time employees working an average of 30 or more hours per week was required to purchase insurance for their employees. Part-time employees were also included. An employer with part-time employees was supposed to report the ratio of the number of hours their part-timers worked a month divided by 120. The answer was considered the number "full-time equivalent" employees. If an employer had 4 part-time employers who work 30 hours a week for a total of 160 hours per month, for example, it had four full-time equivalent employees.[x, 130]

Predictably, the effects of the ACA on businesses were disastrous. First, the trend towards skyrocketing premiums was not reversed. It accelerated. Second, the penalties were insufficient to

[x] (Four employees x 30 hours per week x 4 weeks in a month) ÷ by 120.

motivate likely non-consumers to purchase healthcare insurance, choosing to pay a penalty instead. Third, the government subsidies for insurers were insufficient to control premiums. Fourth, out-of-pocket expenses increased. Fifth, the mandate created by the government regarding benefits reduced insurer flexibility resulting in further price elevations. And finally, the ACA had the secondary effect of incentivizing some businesses to outsource their work to avoid the mandate while others began hiring part-time workers.

The effects on healthcare access were also harsh. Although the number of uninsured in the United States fell to 27 million, a difference of 17 million individuals,[131] 14 million were Medicaid enrollees of whom approximately 3.4 million were already eligible.[132] Thus, only about 11 million new individuals actually became eligible for Medicaid as a result of the ACA.[133] Another 2.3 million of those gaining health insurances were not direct purchasers of healthcare insurance consumers, but rather young adults who became eligible for coverage under their parent's health insurance plan.[134] So, ultimately, the ACA only added 3.8 million individuals as private payer beneficiaries through their own accord, 6.1 million if one includes those covered through their parents' policies;[135] a paltry number indeed.

In effect, what the ACA did was to require every American to purchase healthcare insurance, either through their employer or on their own. The government reasoned that the high concentration of healthcare consumers amongst the insured was a large contributor to the spiraling costs of health insurance. In other words, not enough young, healthy people were voluntarily purchasing health insurance, and too many unhealthy or older people were. If insufficient numbers of healthy people were buying insurance, the solution was to simply pressure them into doing so under the pain of penalty. Those penalties collected from the noncompliant would then be used to subsidize insurance companies that sold government-approved healthcare plans.

The ACA brought with it several constitutional questions. In a government where congressional powers are specifically and finitely enumerated, by what authority was Congress passing this legislation? Did Congress really have the authority to require that a person enter a market even if he or she was not motivated to do so? Were the actions of a person who chose not to participate in the market really covered by the Interstate Commerce Clause? And ultimately, did Congress really have the authority to force someone to purchase healthcare insurance by virtue of the person's birth? This last question would ultimately get posed to the Supreme Court in the case *National Federation of Independent Businesses. v. Sebelius*.[136]

Under even the broadest reading of the Constitution, Congress was not expressly given the authority to require individuals to purchase health insurance. Thus, in order to defend its mandate, the government would have to interpret an implicit power in the Constitution. The proponents of Obamacare argued that this authority existed through the Interstate Commerce Clause. But there was a problem with this argument. The delivery of healthcare to any particular patient does not across state lines since all the actors, patient and healthcare personnel alike, are present in the same room, or at least in the same building.

But the proponents of Obamacare argued they were regulating health insurance, not the actual healthcare interaction, which *did* cross state lines. Recall that under *Wickard*, the Supreme Court had already ruled that Congress could regulate intrastate activities if those activities, *in their aggregate*, impacted interstate commerce. And of course, at 20% of the GDP healthcare and the insurance industry had a major aggregate impact on the national economy.

In the eyes of Congress, premiums were skyrocketing. Employers were finding it difficult to afford health insurance. Patients, many of them employees, were unable to afford their own healthcare coverage, and some were even going bankrupt because of their inability to afford healthcare coverage. For all these reasons, said the interventionist proponents, health insurance needed reform, and it definitely fell within the purview of congressional authority to do so.

But never in the history of the United States had a law forced someone to enter the market if they otherwise refused to do so. The *Wickard* case never addressed Congress's power to force individuals to enter the market (buy health insurance) whether they wanted to or not. Indeed, such a broad interpretation of the Interstate Commerce Clause would allow Congress to coerce people into all sorts of activities they would otherwise have avoided. Conceivably, in the name of health, Congress could force the individual to buy certain foods, enroll in health classes, exercise a minimum period of time each day, and purchase certain equipment. According to the late Justice Antonin Scalia, to allow such an expansive interpretation of federal authority would be "to make mere breathing in and out the basis for federal prescription and to extend power to virtually all human activity."[137]

The implications of Congress's newfound powers would belie every premise Americans had previously held regarding their relationship with government. The notion that Congress could possess such broad powers was so preposterous that even its proponents realized it would not stand up to constitutional scrutiny.

By the time the case reached the Supreme Court, the government was delivering a second theory. It argued the ACA was constitutional because Congress was not relying on the Interstate Commerce Clause as its foundation. Rather, its actions fell within the authorities granted to it under the Tax And Spend Clause. You see, said the government, those fees charged to the people who did not purchase prescribed insurance products were not penalties; they were taxes!

In a 5 to 4 ruling Chief Justice John Roberts writing the opinion for the Court agreed that what was explicitly named "penalties" in the ACA were actually "taxes." And in so doing, the Court forever changed healthcare in America.[138] Chief Justice Roberts said about the mandate to purchase insurance, "[It] is not a legal command to buy insurance. Rather, it makes going without insurance just another thing the government taxes, like buying gasoline or earning an income."[139] His observation is flawed, however, because taxing people for not buying insurance is more akin to the government taxing them for not buying gasoline or not earning an income, which of course, the government has never done.

Justice Scalia's dissent was particularly telling, as his principal concern was the grand expansion of authority afforded to Congress under the Court's majority interpretation. First, he correctly pointed out "abstention from commerce–is not 'Commerce.'"[140] and second, although "*purchasing* insurance *is* 'Commerce'...one does not regulate commerce that does not exist by compelling its existence."[141] Further, in reference to considering the ACA penalties taxes, Scalia pointed out that the two are mutually exclusive. A tax cannot be a penalty for constitutional purposes, nor can a penalty be considered a tax. According to Scalia and the three other justices who joined him in his dissent, the Court had held "that a 'tax' imposed on private conduct was so onerous as to be in effect a penalty.

But [it had] never held–never–that a penalty imposed for violation of the law was so trivial as to be in effect a tax."[142] Even more damning was Scalia's observation that the actual ACA legislation specifically named these fees "penalties," not "taxes," and the Supreme Court "cannot rewrite a statute what it is not."[143] Tragically, this is exactly what the Court did in this case.

The fact that the ACA was allowed to stand serves as a testament not only to the dangers inherent to the growing usurpation of power by the Supreme Court, but also of the dangers posed by a Court that fails to follow the strict interpretations of the law and of the Constitution.

As of this writing, Republicans have unsuccessfully attempted to fully repeal the ACA on substantive grounds. Nevertheless, in 2017, the Tax Cuts and Jobs Act reduced the personal responsibility payments for not having insurance (the penalties/taxes) to zero. Subsequently, a federal court ruled that the absence of an imposed payment rendered the mandate to purchase unconstitutional.[144] The matter is presently under appeal.

Healthcare Manufacturing and Durable Goods Regulation

The impact of government on healthcare under the progressives' agenda has gone way beyond direct interference with the actions of providers. It has touched every facet of the healthcare delivery system, from drug manufacturing to administration, implant production to delivery, food preparation to consumption, and worker hiring to firing. In fewer places has the erected structure of governmental oversight of healthcare been so faulty as in the arena of medications and drug manufacturing.

Quackery, alchemy, and "potionology" have been a part of the United States since its inception. The manufacturing, marketing, and selling of snake oils, charms, and potions by quacks and others presenting themselves as experts on medical conditions predate the nation's foundation. In fact, as touched upon in Chapter 2, the expanded practice by individuals with suspect credentials during the nineteenth century became the source of the first medical malpractice crisis in the United States.

As time went on, advances in chemistry and distribution technology led to the exposure of the public to increasingly dangerous chemicals with broader dispersal bandwidths. Chemist Harvey W. Wiley who served as the head of the United States Department of Agriculture's Division of Chemistry during the 1800s is generally credited with first bringing the dangers of untested products to Congress's attention when a diphtheria antitoxin taken from a tetanus contaminated horse caused the deaths of over a dozen children. In response, Congress passed the Biologic Control Act of 1902 authorizing the regulation of vaccines and anti-toxins.[145]

During the 1920s, Congress continued to dabble in the arena of food and drug regulation, passing, among other statutes, the Pure Food and Drug Act in 1906 (also known as the Wiley Act). Over time, the Division of Chemistry became known as the Food, Drug, and Insecticide Administration and ultimately, in 1930, the Food and Drug Administration (FDA).[146]

But then, in 1937, bacteriologists created an antibiotic named sulfanilamide, which was extremely effective against streptococcal infections, "strep." The manufacturer, the S. E. Massengill Company, recognized the benefits this medicine could have on children who were frequently afflicted with strep infections. Massengill recognized that a liquid form of the medication would be preferable if it was going to be marketed for children's diseases. The S.E. Massengill Company eventually arrived at diethylene glycol as a suitable liquid solvent for the medication and released over 240 gallons of the elixir in September 1937. But the company had not tested the mixture for toxicity prior to releasing it to the public.[147]

Almost immediately, deaths were reported in association with the consumption of the liquid form of sulfanilamide, and Massengill quickly recalled its product. As it turned out, the diethylene glycol used in the liquid form of sulfanilamide was a poisonous compound commonly used in antifreeze and known to the FDA,[148] but the laws of the time did not allow it to readily review the medicine before its release, nor did it allow for the easy assumption of jurisdiction during the investigation. The FDA was ultimately able to assume jurisdiction of the case as a mislabeling event because the drug had incidentally been sold as an elixir despite not containing any alcohol.[149]

Between the FDA's efforts and those of the S. E. Massengill Company, the distributed medications were expeditiously found and the public warned of the drug's dangers, but not before 107 deaths had occurred.[150]

The events surrounding the sulfanilamide crisis served as the call for greater regulatory oversight of the food and drug industry, leading to the Food, Drug, and Cosmetic Act of 1938, which gave rise to the FDA we know it today. Under the 1938 Act, the FDA was given the authority to, among other things, approve any drug deemed "safe and effective" in the treatment of a medical condition.[151] The FDA was also given the authority to approve surgical implants and medical devices before they hit the market. The FDA was not chartered to serve as a great coordinating agency for future research in medicine or to fill in any gaps in our pharmacological armamentarium and our medical needs. Instead, such innovative ventures were left in the hands of the private sector.

Since its inception, the FDA has grown into a colossal government organization with a budget of $5.116 billion per year[152] and given direct oversight responsibilities over a segment of the American economy accounting for up to 25% of the gross domestic product, or over $1 trillion annually.[153] In so doing, the FDA has developed an intense and progressively involved process through which a new drug or device is allowed in the market.

When an inventor (referred to by the FDA as a sponsor) desires to bring a drug or medical device to the consumer, its first goal is to demonstrate that the product is a sage and effective treatment for the targeted medical condition. The sponsor must demonstrate that the drug is safe for human testing. This is usually done through animal testing. Once the sponsor believes that the medication or device is safe for human testing, it may submit an Investigational New Drug Application (IND) complete with its objective support of the drug's safety in humans. If the FDA agrees that the drug is safe for human trialing, the sponsor may begin designing its prospective Phase 1 trial. During this phase, the drug is usually administered to between 20 and 80 healthy volunteers with the sole aim of identifying side effects and to better define its metabolism and pharmacology. The emphasis during Phase I testing is safety.

If the drug successfully passes through Phase 1, it may then move to Phase 2 where its effectiveness against the condition being treated is examined. During this second phase of testing, the number of human subjects increases, and even though safety continues to be evaluated, the primary concern shifts to performance. This is classically where the treatment outcomes are compared to placebos or other standards.

The medication or device, if preliminarily found to be safe and effective, may then undergo Phase 3 testing where more rigorous clinical testing is undertaken, all under the guidance of the FDA. The number of people studied during the Phase 3 portions of the trial may amount to hundreds or thousands.

Only after the drug passes phase 3 testing may it be approved for marketing, and even still, this approval is tantamount to a provisional one where the FDA plays an active role in defining the post-market requirements and commitment studies on the part of the sponsor. At this point, the sponsor may file a New Drug Application (NDA) replete with all applicable animal and human data and their analyses. The FDA then has 60 days to decide whether to file the application with the Center for Drug Evaluation and Research (CDER), which must act on at least 90% of the NDAs within ten months of their receipt.[154]

For decades, the FDA has faced criticisms regarding its policies and procedures. For example, under the present structure, the typical drug approval process costs about $1.2 billion.[155] As would be expected, some of this cost is due to the necessary care required to demonstrate the safety and efficacy of a product. There was a time the FDA would take over two years to review a prospective drug, most of the delays being due to chronic backlogs within the agency.[156] Facing pressure from Congress and consumers alike to accelerate and streamline its drug approval process, the FDA cut down its lag time to about 18 months during the 1990s.[157] But in 2014, its efforts were brought to task when a novel non-steroidal anti-inflammatory medication it had approved, Vioxx, resulted in a higher incidence of strokes and heart attacks than controls.[158]

Wounded by the experience, the FDA returned to a slower approval process that resulted in a 25% decline in turn around time[159] and significant variability in the productivities of its various departments. For example, presently, the slowest division, the Neurology Division, takes about 600 days to approve or reject medications while the Oncology and Anti-Viral Divisions take only about 200 days.[160] Such differences cannot be explained by the complexity of the medications being reviewed, the division's workload, or diminutions in safety.[161] The study also found that if the slower divisions could narrow the productivity gap by about half, the resulting savings in drug development costs would amount to $800 million annually.[162]

Inefficiencies within the FDA are particularly detrimental since technological advances have made it possible to bring new and previously unimaginable medications to the market at less than 1/100,000 the price of merely eight years ago.[163] Additionally, the staggering costs of the new drug and medical product application process are stymying competition at a time when smaller and leaner manufacturers could be entering it.

Other governmental control factors are suppressing the development of a robust, competitive drug market. As of this writing, 225 medications are found in the American Society of Health-System Pharmacists drug shortages list.[164] Generic injectable medications make up the overwhelming number of these.[165] Essential medications like sodium chloride, the basic solutions making up intravenous fluids, injectable antibiotics like ciprofloxacin, local analgesics like Lidocaine (the most common numbing medicine), and generic cancer drugs abound in the list. The reasons for these shortages point straight at government.

The Medicare Modernization Act (MMA) of 2003 aimed to accomplish with medications what the Balanced Budget Act of 1997 did with provider reimbursements. Progressive legislators and policymakers tried to solve the problem of high drug costs by implementing a mandatory price formula. Under the MMA, medicines in the outpatient setting could only be sold for the average selling price plus six percent and then only increased by six percent semiannually.[166] But the mandate caused significant problems. Following the expiration of its patent, the price of a medication can fall as much as 90%.[167] The patenting drug manufacturers tend to discontinue the production of those medications that have lost their patents. Whereas under normal circumstances, other suppliers would step in to fill the voids created by these absent manufacturers, the incentive for competing manufacturers to enter the market is low under the MMA. Consequently, as the original manufacturers stop making a drug, very few if any competitors step in, leading to the predictable drug shortages.[168]

Adding to this problem is the influence of group purchasing organizations (GPOs). These entities developed within the medical industry to broker the sale of equipment and medications to providers. Under ideal conditions, GPOs contract with manufacturers for discounts in exchange for access to their purchasing members. For example, a GPO controlling the purchases of a certain medication by fifteen hospitals is in a position to negotiate deep discounts for those medications in exchange for the manufacturer's ability to sell its product to the fifteen hospitals the GPO represents. In the United States, networking with GPOs has been a popular practice amongst hospitals. However, these GPO-controlled-networks have grown so large that only the bigger manufacturers have been able to supply the large volumes of products demanded by the GPOs. Additionally, in a market dominated by GPOs, it becomes exceedingly difficult for competitors to enter the market unless it can provide a similar volume of products. Thus, three or fewer manufacturers produced 90%

of all generic injectable oncology medications in the United States in 2010.[169] One would think that artificially strengthening GPOs' positions would be counterintuitive under these circumstances, yet that is exactly what the government has done through federal safe harbor provisions.

The Social Security Act generally prohibits payments exceeding 3% of the sale price in return for purchases or orders made by any private entity participating in a federal healthcare program. Interestingly, and almost inexplicably, GPOs selling to hospitals have been granted an exception to the Social Security Act's anti-kickback statute.[170] GPOs and their clients have therefore engaged in an elaborate scheme of money flow where everyone wins except the patient.

The way this scheme works is as follows. The customer (in this case the hospital), in coordination with a GPO, purchases a product from a vendor. The hospital pays the vendor the reduced price negotiated by the GPO. The vendor then pays a percentage of the proceeds to the GPO. The GPO is then free to send a portion of the proceeds back to the hospital while using the remainder of its fees to fund other products or services.[171] This practice has disseminated so widely that, in 2012 alone, the "administrative fees" collected by the top five GPOs amounted to $2.3 billion![172]

Whether it be Medicare, with its fee or performance mandate induced physician shortages, Medicaid with its pricing limitations, the Affordable Care Act with its failed attempts at reducing premiums and out-of-pocket expenses, or the FDA with its suppressive effects on innovation and drug supplies the overall pattern of government's manipulations on the nation's healthcare system has been less than stellar and often harmful. While limited regulatory governmental oversight for the purposes of ensuring safety and promoting public health is necessary, the consequences of excess regulatory interference are as detrimental to healthcare as they are to any other industry.

Despite calls from the left and uneducated populists for increased regulations and centralized controls, the obvious answers to our healthcare challenges lie in a direction away from government. Countless solutions that do not involve government intervention exist for the problems challenging our healthcare and our nation. These solutions will spur innovation, increase productivity, and most importantly, improve our access to quality, comprehensive and compassionate medical attention. They are necessarily solutions that will take away control from the government and place it squarely in the hands of the consumer.

Government Takes Control over America's Specialty Organizations

The latter half of the twentieth century saw government overpower the judgment and priorities of physician medical organizations, the prime advocates for independence in the practice of medicine. For over a century, the AMA has been the principal organization representing physician interests before government and the public. The AMA advocates for everything from state licensure issues to physician labor, ostensibly on behalf of its members. That same AMA has served as the principal source for education and training material for the nation's physicians. It is therefore imperative that the AMA be beholden to its members and free of any confounding outside influences. But since the latter half of the twentieth century, the AMA's fiduciary relationship to its members has not remained so pure.

In 1965, with the creation of Medicare, government needed to retain the support of the nation's physicians. The AMA, fearing the socialist precepts of the Medicare program, was highly skeptical. It had already vehemently opposed Medicare's original incarnation designed to provide healthcare coverage to all American workers and their families. Among other concerns, the AMA feared that a government-run national reimbursement organization would infringe on how much physicians earned for their services. Consequently, in an effort to satisfy organized medicine, policymakers made sure the proposed Medicare system would provide payments based on very squishy "usual, customary, and reasonable rates."[173] Medicare, of course, was going to pass with or without the backing of America's physicians.

But problems quickly developed. First, a communication system was needed to define the services performed by providers and the conditions for which those services had been administered. And who better to create such a communication system than the principal organization representing the nation's physicians? The AMA quickly went to work to create a new and comprehensive medical language made up of numerical codes. One system, the International Classification of Diseases (ICD codes) was adapted from a nineteenth-century set of codes developed in France. It identified illnesses and supporting ancillary data such as causes of diseases and other epidemiological factors. The other, the Current Procedural Terminology codes (CPT codes), was created by the AMA de novo and was designed to designate the procedures being performed by physicians.

But of course, such a mammoth system of procedural codes and communications technology could not be created for free. Designers, crafters, coding and policy experts, economists, epidemiologists, and yes, physicians needed to be assembled in creating such a comprehensive, technical, and innovative product. And even after the coding system was developed, maintenance and updates needed to be made to accommodate technological advancements and coding gaps. Additionally, once the ICD and CPT codes were structured, a work value had to be attached to each of the listed services. And once again the AMA was tasked with bringing the system, called Relative Value Units (RVUs) to fruition. Thus, the RVU was born. The project became so massive that in 2010, the AMA received $72 million for its production and maintenance.[174] These payments dwarfed the $38 million the AMA received from its membership dues.[175]

Predictably, as the AMA became more dependent on government-generated income, its negotiating abilities against the government began to weaken. Increasingly, the AMA acted as the government's partner more than it did a physician's fiduciary. This intimacy between the government and the AMA may explain how it ended up offering its support to the ACA even though the bill failed to address many of the issues affecting the practice of medicine and negatively impacted its members. The ACA did not correct how physicians were reimbursed, nor did it do away with the then-governing sustainable growth rate (SGR), the flawed and unfair formula dictating how much physicians got paid for their services. In fact, the ACA worsened physician reimbursement because it shuffled money away from Medicare and pushed patients into government-run insurance products, which paid physicians about 14% less than private payers.[176] For the AMA to support the ACA despite its deleterious effect upon its members defies comprehension.

So why did the AMA support the ACA?

The AMA argued its support was based on the prospect of increasing healthcare coverage for the nation's uninsured. It claimed that the plan would make it more difficult for sicker patients to lose their coverage. The AMA also heralded a $245 billon promise it received from government officials that Congress would permanently correct the SGR, which at the time was the medical profession's greatest headache. But in politics more so than in business, a promise based on a handshake is worth only the paper on which it is written.

For years, the AMA did not get the fruits of its naiveté, and when it did, it was given something even worse. It was given the Medicare Access and CHIP Reauthorization Act of 2015 (MACRA), which as a reimbursement scheme functioned even more oppressively than the SGR because it did not increase physician reimbursement for Medicare services and tied payments to computer-based performance measures that became the biggest source of physician frustration and early burnout.

So why would the largest physician professional organization, one with a lobbying arsenal totaling $756.3 million agree to such a disadvantageous deal for its physicians without any concrete solutions to the problems afflicting its members? The answer remains hidden in a murky sea of explanations and excuses, but one thing is certain, it is very difficult to argue against someone or something willing to pay $78 million for services it created for you and then shielded you from having others intrude upon your exclusive right to deliver them.

Government Takes Control of Medical Education and Healthcare Sciences

The federal government's tentacles of influence over medical organizations extend much deeper than mere physician advocacy.

It reaches into the heart of what is taught and sold to our nation's doctors. Once again, the latter half of the twentieth century, with the Herculean growth of the federal government's footprint on society and industry, was the time when government intrusion into the type and magnitude of information provided to physicians blossomed.

To become a doctor, a prospective physician, upon completing his or her baccalaureate education, must enroll in medical school. As of 2012, there were 175 medical colleges[177] with 91,391 medical students.[178] Additionally, there were 26,981 osteopathic enrolled students.[179] Although the number of medical schools is not predetermined, for an institution of medical education to qualify for federal funding and for their graduates to be eligible for eventual licensure in most states, it must be accredited by the Liaison Committee on Medical Education (LCME), the United States Department of Education's accrediting body for programs leading to degrees in either osteopathic and medical doctorates. The LCME's accreditation must then be maintained through compliance with the requirements it sets forth.[180] Incidentally, the LCME is sponsored by the Association of American Medical Colleges (AAMC) and that other pseudo-branch of the federal government, the AMA.[181]

Everything about these teaching institutions is regulated by the LCME inclusive of such mundane components as the composition of the school's leadership team, their academic and learning environments, the presence of diversity programs, their anti-discrimination policies, their financial resources, their security measures, their library and information technology, their curricula, and their medical student selection processes, to name a few.[182] The federal government, through its proxies, has thus taken control of the design and maintenance of those institutions responsible for the genesis of the nation's medical caregivers and keepers.[183]

Once the young physician graduates from medical school, training intensity increases dramatically as he or she undertakes the most trying portion of his or her medical education: his or her internship, residency, and fellowship training. This process, collectively called the doctor's postgraduate training, is also deeply imprinted with the ink of federal oversight and influence. In 2015, over $14.5 billion of American tax dollars were spent in support of residency and fellowship training, with more than 90% of those dollars coming from Medicare and Medicaid.[184] Through its influence in the postgraduate process, the federal government expressly aims to correct mismatches between the health needs of a population and its perceived distribution of physicians, shortcomings in the diversity of the physician population, gaps between the knowledge physicians take into the workplace and those the government believes those physicians need to possess, and any perceived lack of fiscal transparency.[185] Of course, these goals and their appropriateness lie virtually unevaluated by the general population since it isn't even aware that its government is engaged in these activities.

All these interactions result in a massive influence from government on the knowledge a young physician takes with him or her to tackle disease. And this undue governmental influence continues for the rest of the doctor's career. One classic scenario of how this works has played itself out in the arena of breast cancer prevention.

In the United States, about 12% of women develop invasive breast cancer. In 2019 alone, there were approximately 268,600 new invasive cases, 62,930 new non-invasive cases, and 41,760 deaths.[186] Because breast cancer is so inconsistently cured, the principal effort at preventing breast-cancer-related deaths is early detection.

Initial efforts at early detection were centered on self-examination. Women were instructed to perform breast self- examinations once a month (using the arrival of the electric bill as a reminder, for example) with the aim of detecting new or unusual lumps in their breasts. Unfortunately, not only did such efforts suffer from inconsistency in compliance, but also the wide variety of breast densities and even density variations within a woman's gestational cycle made the exercise quite ineffective. Predictably, women were presenting to their doctors with reports of what turned out to be benign lesions while others were missing the diagnosis of malignancy entirely.

Technological advances allowed for the use of mammography to become the principal method for the early detection of suspicious breast lesions. These low-intensity x-rays allowed pictures to be taken through a woman's breasts facilitating the identification of suspicious lesions. The lesions could then be biopsied for definitive diagnoses as benign or malignant growths.

Although much more effective at identifying early cancerous lesions than the breast self-examination, mammography still suffered from inaccuracies and complications. First, the interpretations of the pictures were often subjective and dependent on a trained human eye to determine whether a lesion was worthy of being biopsied or not. This uncertainty was exacerbated by the denseness of the underlying breast tissue, and since younger women have denser breasts, they were particularly prone to experiencing erroneous mammograms with falsely positive results.

The radiation associated with mammograms was also a concern. This, combined with the lower incidence of breast cancer in younger women, made recommending mammography in young women unfavorable. The competing priorities between the desire to save women's lives through the early detection and avoidance of unnecessary procedures and their complications led to a balancing act in determining the best approach for mammography. If the recommendation was too aggressive, women were going to be unnecessarily exposed to pain, suffering, expense, worry, and confusion. Too lax, and women would die.

Various medical groups studied the issue and published their opinions regarding the best ways of detecting the appearance of breast cancer. Initial recommendations were that women undergo baseline mammography at some point between the ages of 35 and 40 years of age followed by yearly mammograms beginning at age 40. Some recommended biennial mammograms in women between 40 and 50 years of age followed by yearly mammograms for those 51 and older. And presently, the National Comprehensive Cancer Network, the American Congress of Obstetricians and Gynecologist, and the American College of Radiology each recommend yearly mammographic screening for breast cancer starting at 40 years of age.[187]

Enter the federal government and the United States Preventive Services Task Force (USPSTF). The USPSTF is a "volunteer panel of national experts in prevention and evidence-based medicine"[188] created in 1984 by the United States Public Health Service.[189] Originally, its purpose was to provide "evidence-based recommendations about clinical preventive services and health promotion."[190] Generally, the USPSTF provides approval or disapproval of certain preventive services and procedures by assigning each a grade. An "A" or "B" grade meant that the practice had sufficient scientific support in the panel's opinion to recommend that the service be offered to the public.[191] Grade "C," "D," or "I" recommendations carried varied implications, but shared a commonality in the lack of enthusiasm for it by the USPSTF.[192]

In 2002, in keeping with the prevailing positions of the nation's leading physician organizations, the USPSTF awarded a B grade to the recommendation that women 40 years old and older should undergo mammography every one to two years.[193]

That changed in 2009.

The table below allows for the direct comparison regarding mammography recommendations from the USPSTF and other medical groups. Although biennial mammography was awarded a B grade in women 50 to 74 years of age, a C grade was given to the practice of routinely performing screening mammograms in women aged 40 to 49 years.[194] In contraposition to the opinions of most national physician and patient organizations, the USPSTF did not support mammography in 40 to 50-year-old women and abandoned the practice of screening women older than 74 years of age. In defending its position to abandon screening of women in their fifth decade of life, the USPSTF simply and offensively averred, "While screening mammography in women aged 40 to 49 years may reduce the risk of breast cancer death, the number of deaths averted is smaller than that in older women and the number of false-positive results and unnecessary biopsies is larger."[195] But in 2017 alone, 49,360 thousand women between the ages of 40-and 49 years were diagnosed with breast cancer (36,920 of those invasive) and 3,480 women in that age group died from it.[196] These are women at the height of their productivity who were raising families and making invaluable contributions to society.

The USPSTF's change in recommendations regarding women aged 75 and older is just as perplexing since the risk of developing breast cancer is known to increase exponentially with age. The chances of developing breast cancer in women between 70 and 80 years of age are one in 26.[197] Moreover, in 2017, there were 92,070 new cases of breast cancer (77,940 of them invasive) and 19,130 deaths in women who were 75 years of age or older (see table on the following pages).

If it weren't for the ACA, however, this would only be a story about internal disagreements among physician groups. But in a move screaming of unconstitutionality, Congress included a provision within the ACA requiring insurers to cover any preventive services awarded a grade of A or B by the USPSTF without copays or deductibles.[198] It also gave the SecHHS, the authority to allow Medicare to cover preventive measures only if they carried an A or B rating from the USPSTF.[199] In light of the USTPSF's decisions, many insurers opted to no longer cover mammography in 40 to 50 year-olds, and Medicare discontinued its coverage for mammograms in women 75 years of age and older.

Why did Congress pick the USPSTF's position as the "official" harbinger of recommendations regarding preventive health over the other professional groups? Because the USPSTF is part of the machinery of government. It is an official government agency, and therefore the legislature could reasonably conclude that it ought to serve as the official voice of the federal government on issues of disease prevention.

Suddenly, the panel of "volunteers" serving on the USPSTF went from being a relatively obscure group delivering just another set of opinions on how the nation should approach its preventive medicine efforts to being the object of intense lobbying efforts by a variety of interests with millions of dollars at stake.[200, 201]

Figure 3-2: Recommendations for Screening Mammograms

Physician Organization	Women Aged 40-49	Women Aged 50-74	Women Aged 75 or Older
United States Preventive Services Task Force 2016[a]	Individual decision for biennial screening mammograms	Biennial screening mammograms	Insufficient evidence. Mammography not recommended
American Cancer Society 2015[b]	Yearly mammograms beginning at age 45	Yearly mammograms for women aged 50-54; women aged 55 and older should either continue with yearly or switch to biennial screening mammograms	Screening mammograms should stop when life expectancy is less than 10 years based on age or comorbid conditions
American College of Obstetrics and Gynecology 2011[c]	Yearly screening mammograms and clinical breast exams	Yearly screening mammograms and clinical breast exams	Mammography optional
International Agency for Research and Cancer 2015[d]	Screening mammograms not recommended	Yearly mammograms recommended for women aged 50-69 years. The benefit of mammography is recognized, but without formal recommendation	Not addressed by this agency
American College of Radiology 2010[e]	Yearly mammograms beginning at age 40	Yearly screening mammograms	Screening mammograms should stop when life expectancy is less than 5-7 years based on age or comorbid conditions

American College of Physicians[f]	Individual decision for biennial mammograms	Biennial screening mammograms	Mammography not recommended
American Academy of Family Physicians 2016[g]	Individual decision	Biennial screening mammograms	Insufficient evidence

[a] A.L Siu, Screening for Breast Cancer; U.S. Preventive Services Task Force Recommendation Statement," Annals of Internal Medicine, 2016; (164):279-296.

[b] K. C. Oeffinger, E. T. Fontham, et al., "Breast Cancer Screening for Women at Average Risk: 2015 Guideline Update from the American Cancer Society," JAMA, 2015;314(15):1599-1614.

[c] American College of Obstetricians-Gynecology, "Practice Bulletin No. 122: Breast Cancer Screening, Obstetrics and Gynecology 2011;118(2 Pt 1):372-382

[d] B. Lauby-Secretan, D. loomis, and K. Straif, "Breast Cancer Screening-Viewpoint of the IARC Working Group," New England Journal of Medicine, 2015;373(15):1478-1479.

[e] C. H. Lee, D. D. Dershaw, et al., "Breast Cancer Screening with Imaging: Recommendations from the Society of Breast Imaging and the ACR on the USe of Mammography, Breast MRI, Breast Ultrasound, and Other Techniques for the Detection of Clinically Occult Breast Cancer," Journal of the American College of Radiology, 2010;7(1):18-27.

[f] T. J. Wilt, R. P. Harris, et al., "Screening for Cancer: Advice for High-Value Care from the American College of Physicians," Annals of Internal Medicine, 2015;162(10):718-725.

[g] American Academy of Family Physician, "Summary of Recommendations for Clinical Preventive Services. July 2017," accessed on Feb. 1, 2020, https://www.aafp.org/dam/AAFP/documents/patient_care/clinical_recommendations/cps-recommendations.pdf.

And just who are these volunteers? They are a group of sixteen "members who are nationally recognized experts in prevention, evidence-based medicine, and primary care...with expertise in behavioral health, family medicine, geriatrics, internal medicine, pediatrics, obstetrics and gynecology, and nursing."[202] For the record, thirteen of the sixteen members are physicians.[203] These members are assigned by the Director of the Agency for Healthcare Research and Quality,[204] who, in turn, is appointed by the SecHHS.[205] So, although the USPSTF likes to think of itself as a scientific, apolitical group, the fact that it is composed of members whose assignments can be traced back to a hierarchy ending at the President of the United States negates that view.

Predictably, the USPSTF's decision to not affirmatively recommend screening mammograms for women in their fifth decades of life and for those older than 74 was fraught with controversy, particularly in light of the newly created funding and access implications the decision carried. The fallout from the recommendations was so bad that Congress overruled it, first temporarily and then, in 2015, permanently.[206] And although Congress can nullify the effects of the USPSTF decision as it relates to Medicare, its authority does not extend to private insurers such that nonfederal programs are still free to honor USPSTF's 2009 recommendations. Incidentally, in its obstinacy, the USPSTF reaffirmed its 2009 recommendations in 2016.

The story of the USPSTF and mammography brings up a number of issues regarding the interplay between government and medicine. First is the overarching question we have previously visited regarding the pinnacle of a democratic state's authority. Is it we the people who stand at that pinnacle with government at our service, or is it government that crowns it? If government is allowed to take its place at the apex, then it is totally appropriate for it to determine what interventions are appropriate for the sake of prolonging our lives and which are not. Can one have a mammogram, and if so at what age? When is someone no longer allowed to have a mammogram? Should they even be tested? These questions may validly fall upon government only if it were the ultimate purveyor of power, and we, its servants.

If, however, each human being has an inestimable value and government exists to facilitate the peaceful coexistence of men, then the concept of government deciding whose life to prolong and whose not is nonsensical and unacceptable.

We may question how it is that things progressed to such an extent that Congress felt compelled to intercede. But it was Congress that created this mess in the first place. Until the Obama Administration, with the Democrats' zeal to centralize healthcare, the USPSTF was a mere think tank, albeit one under the umbrella of the fourth branch of government, but still, a mere think tank. Whether the federal government should even be running such a think tank is subject to debate, but regardless, before 2010 and certainly in 2009 when the USPSTF's position on mammography became more restrictive, its opinion on mammography was simply that, an opinion. It was not until Congress decided to dictate healthcare prevention policy through one of its agencies that things went awry.

Also, consider how deeply enmeshed within the recesses of bureaucratic layers the USPSTF is. This is an agency whose members are appointed by a Director, who is himself *appointed* by a Secretary who is appointed by the President of the United States. At least three levels of unaccountability exist between the American people and the persons making decisions on preventive medicine resources, with each level cloaked in increasing anonymity.

Who are the actual members of the USPSTF? From what parts of the country do they proceed? What are their political views and inclinations? What are their philosophies on government and its role in healthcare? The public does not know the answers to these questions, yet those individuals are the ones making life and death decisions for our nation.

Their apologists claim this is not a political body, as it is made up of scientists. But here, the observations made by Thomas Jefferson regarding judges are equally as applicable to the members of the USPSTF: "[They] are as honest as other men, and not more so. They have, with others, the same passions for party, for power, and the privilege of their corps. . . and their power the more dangerous as they are...not responsible, as the other functionaries are, to the elective control."[207]

The fact is that each of us carries philosophical views on the relationship between man and government. These views may mature. They may grow and morph into shapes and colors that they had never previously possessed. But regardless of their form and contents, they shape our opinions and our decisions. Any time one says, "the government should do this," or "the government ought never meddle," one is expressing a political opinion. And if one is given the privilege of shaping policy, the moment one allows his or her recommendations to shape government action, even if functioning as an "expert" or "scientist," one necessarily injects his or her political views into the discussion.

Suppose, as an expert, you conclude that outlawing 32-ounce sodas may improve the nation's obesity problem. Indeed, every expert in the field of 32-ounce "sodaology" may agree with you, but the moment you recommend outlawing 32-ounce sodas, you have injected your political views into the matter. As an expert, you could have acknowledged the basic truism in sodaology regarding the unhealthiness of 32-ounce sodas, but you could have concluded, while still maintaining your allegiance to your field, that outlawing 32-ounce drinks is not an appropriate governmental action. Both positions are based on the premise that drinking 32-ounce sodas is unhealthy, but one view is informed by an expansive view of government, and the other by a minimalist one. There is no in-between.

In some ways, this dynamic leads to a self-fulfilling prophecy in governance. If you happened to be the expert opining that regulating 32-ounce sodas does not fall within the role of government, your chances of getting appointed to a board designed to regulate 32-ounce sodas are dramatically less. On the other hand, if you are a vociferous advocate of such policies, the moment the pro-regulatory majority gains power, you're in! A non-interventionist majority will not create a board designed to study whether it is a good idea to abstain from regulating 32-ounce sodas, as it has no interest in passing such regulation. But a pro-regulatory majority will with the opposite intent, and when it does, it will not appoint an opponent to such regulatory interventions, but rather, a fellow expansionist. Thus in government, it is the expansionists that tend to get hired to make commentaries about passing restrictive legislation, not the restrictionists for opining that government does not.

Finally, there is the inherent contradiction of having Congress intervene in a decision made by one of its agencies. By its very assignment of a matter to an agency, Congress has acknowledged that it does not possess the expertise or the political will to handle the matter directly. If it did, Congress itself would have passed the necessary law.

So what does it say about Congress that after it handed the ball on a matter to an unelected band of experts it should have to overrule it? Do we believe it appropriate for Congress to be deciding whether any one of us ought to be ineligible for mammography as an insurance benefit? Yet this situation, and hundreds of thousands like it, would flourish if we adopt a government-run system of healthcare.

Hospital Regulation as a Vehicle for Controlling Healthcare Delivery

The most effective location to regulate doctors in mass quantities is the hospital. Hospitals are corporate entities. They are not advocates for medicine. They have little stake in the politics of the medical profession and in the art of medicine. In carrying out their functions, theirs is to comply with the legislative environment in which they exist. When an overseeing federal agency mandates that they change the way their physicians practice medicine, hospitals do not generally complain. They do not demand to view the literature supporting the new mandate or ask by what method that regulation was made. They especially do not challenge the scientific merits of the mandate. Instead, they enact policies that implement the changes imposed upon them by the government.

The government's recurring and seemingly senseless interventions on pain control are great examples of the complex interplay between government, hospitals, physicians, and the negative consequences such forays may carry.

In an effort to stem the tide of the nation's ongoing opioid crisis, the government has sought to manipulate how your doctor manages your pain during your hospitalization. Let's say it's 1992 and you've just had a hip replacement and are wheeled back from the recovery room to your room. You're in horrific pain; pain so bad you're writhing in it. Your nurse already knows a little bit about your surgery and you because she has just gotten off the phone with your post-anesthesia care unit nurse who gave her a report about you, the surgery you just had, the fluids you're receiving, your vital signs, the doctor's plans for you, and the medications you have just received. What your nurse does not know about you until now is what you look like and the kind of discomfort you're in. In fact, this is the first opportunity she has to formulate a direct impression of the type of pain you're in.

As you're being wheeled into the room, the floor nurse asks you how much pain you're in on a scale of one through ten. You respond with a ten.

But there are tens, and then there are tens. And yours is real ten!

This particular nurse happens to have been practicing in this very ward for over a decade where your doctor has been performing surgery for just as long. She has seen thousands of hip replacement patients at the very same stage of recovery as yours, and having worked with your doctor as she has, she is just as familiar with your surgeon's style and preferences.

As is her duty, she evaluates you. She takes your vital signs. She looks at the dressings. She assesses your hip and your leg and examines you thoroughly. She concludes you need a dose of morphine because an oral analgesic will not control your pain. She combs through your chart to find your medication orders. She finds an order for three milligrams of morphine to be administered through your veins or injected into your muscle every three hours, as needed, for pain. Below the morphine order, there's another order for oxycodone, an oral narcotic analgesic, also to be administered as needed for pain.

From her vast experience, she can tell that your pain will overwhelm the effects of the oxycodone. She also knows that you need fast relief. She decides intravenous morphine is the way to go for you. She goes to the floor's medication dispensary, and while witnessed, retrieves a prepackaged dose of morphine for you. Moments later, she returns to your room, vial in hand, and administers your pain medication, affording you the relief you needed.

But things have changed since 1992. Back then physician orders were recorded holographically, and like today, some pain medication orders were written to be activated if a certain range of conditions existed. In the early 90s, the range triggering pain severities were classified as "mild," "moderate," and "severe." For example, your doctor might say that the staff should give you Tylenol for mild pain, one tablet of hydrocodone for moderate pain, or a Percocet tablet for severe pain. The severity of the pain, like its descriptors, was subjective, as pain severity by definition is.

Even back then, some ascribed numbers to the pain ("How bad is it on a scale of one through ten?"), but that number, whether documented or not, was used as a supplement to an overall, subjective assessment of the intensity of the patient's pain. Based on this overall impression, superimposed on the nurse's experience, a decision would be made as to the most appropriate medication you should receive.

With the advent of computers, range orders became more specific. Words were exchanged for numbers and nurse discretion was removed. Soon government would inject itself into this complex and necessarily subjective interplay between physician, nurse, and patient with devastating public health effects. The events leading to this tragic case of governmental interference began in 1995 when the American Pain Society floated the idea that pain should be considered the fifth vital sign, joining blood pressure, pulse, breathing rate, and temperature as the other four.[208, 209] Its goal was to raise awareness of the under-treatment of pain.

But in 2000, the federal government felt the need to get involved through the Joint Commission (JCO), the organization chartered with the responsibility of overseeing hospitals participating in Medicare. That year, JCO published an Element of Performance (EP), or a standard by which hospitals were to be judged and expected to meet. The standard, known as RI. 1.1.8, read that the patient had a "right to pain management [that needed to be] respected and supported."[210] Hospitals were required to hand out pain management informational packets stating, among other things, "Your report of your pain *will be believed.*"[211] (Emphasis added.)

The following year, JCO (then known as JCAHO) published another rule called EP 1.4, requiring that "[p]ain [be] assessed on all patients."[212] In its explanation, JCO recommended that a numerical scale or an emotional-face-scale be employed to allow the patient to communicate the severity of his or her pain.[xi, 213]

The publication of the new rule signaled that JCO would be evaluating hospitals in its periodic inspections to make sure they were implementing these new requirements. Compliance was required if a hospital was to maintain its accreditation with Medicare. Additionally, the hospital's compliance score would be published, which could either be employed as a boasting point by a hospital if good, or published by the local newspapers to shame it if not.

[xi] An emotional-face scale is a figure demonstrating a series of cartoon faces correlating with a number on a scale, usually one through ten. The emotion depicted on each face suggests the level of discomfort correlating with the number on a scale. It is used to assist patients in communicating the intensity of their pain.

But things got even dicier when JCO published a book on pain management sponsored by Purdue Pharma, a principal manufacturer of pain medications, directed at physicians.[214] Chief amongst these medications was Oxycontin, a slow-release form of oxycodone. All over the country, attractive sales representatives bought lunches for physicians and their staffs and presented them with data, produced by the manufacturer, demonstrating the safety and efficacy of their product while touting their exceedingly low addiction rates.[215] The result was a monumental expansion in the use of narcotic medications within the United States. Healthcare personnel, physicians and nurses alike, driven to an obsessive preoccupation with pain scores by government, pushed narcotics medications upon their patients to make sure the "fifth vital sign" was maintained at controlled levels. Subsequently, 385,757 people died of drug overdoses in the United States between 2001 and 2017 while millions more suffered from addiction.[216, 217]

So, is government policy responsible for the explosion of opioid overuse and abuse? It certainly has a hand in it.

The truth is the opioid epidemic afflicting Americans is multi-factorial. Broken families, moral apathy, drug pushers seeking to make a profit, manufacturers overly and unethically encouraging providers to prescribe pain medications, physicians overprescribing (some seeking the profits of illegal pill mills) are all factors causing the mess in which we find ourselves. But any neutral observer must acknowledge that a government policy promoting the obsession of maximum pain relief implemented by individuals having no knowledge of the nuances of taking care of patients necessarily played a role in kick-starting the present crisis.

Even a cursory look at the opioid overdose death curve reveals the massive acceleration in the mortality ascribable to opioids that started in 2001, the same year JCO began implementing and enforcing its pain management policies. In 2000, for example, there were 8,407 deaths from an opioid overdose, about the same number as years past. By 2010, the number increased to 21,088, and in 2017, the number of opioid-related deaths in a single year had risen to 47,600.[218] How interesting that the precipitous increase in opioid deaths began the very year that JCO intervened on provider's pain relief practices!

In 2009, JCO did what it should have done from the very beginning. It removed its standard to assess pain in all patients. But its withdrawal from pain management regulation was short-lived as the agency reinstated a pain management EP in 2018 after "conducting an extensive literature review on contemporary clinical guidelines and best practices for pain assessment and management, including safe opioid prescribing."[219] Ostensibly having learned its lesson regarding the direct imposition of its will on the practice of medicine, JCO placed the onus on hospitals to create leadership teams "responsible for pain management and safe opioid prescribing."[220]

The fact is that these regulatory interventions are not esoteric discussion points since they have direct and palpable effects on how you get your healthcare. All we have to do is revisit the perioperative pain control events we reviewed earlier in this chapter.

Suppose that like before, you are writhing in pain following your hip replacement surgery and are being taken care of by the ten-year veteran nurse as you are wheeled to your hospital room. Only this time, the year is 2020.

Upon completing her initial assessment, your nurse asks you to report how bad your pain is, and you answer, "Really bad." Patiently, she asks you to give her a number on a scale of one through ten with 0 being no pain and 10 being the worst pain you could imagine. To help you, she pulls out a little emotional-pain-scale so you may better communicate your pain assessment to her.

Flippantly, you bark, "Twelve!" She responds by informing you that she is going to document it as a ten because her electronic medical records do not allow her to input twelve.

She then turns to her electronic tablet in search of the pain medication orders. Once again, she *knows* a dose of morphine is the most appropriate for you, but the orders are pretty explicit as required by your hospital's JCO-implemented Pain Management Committee. Your doctor can no longer write for Morphine *and* oxycodone for "severe pain." Now, because of the unyielding software and in compliance with the rules of the Committee, he must write the orders based on pain scores *and* must denote which medication he wants you to have first.

Of course, your doctor is not at your bedside to actually evaluate you as you ask for pain medication, but nurses are no longer regulatorily entrusted to make judgments on the patient's pain severity despite their extensive, training, and experience.[xii] Consequently, the physician must now specify the actual dose to be administered *prospectively*. Additionally, your doctor can no longer write a strength range for your medications. Where he used to be able to tell your nurse to administer 2 to 4 milligrams of morphine every four hours as needed for severe pain, your doctor must now state the exact dose to be given, the numerical pain scale for which it must be given, and which medication is to be administered first when range orders overlap.

[xii] Recall that the same policymakers stating that nurses are not to be trusted in deciphering the medication strength to be administered in response to a patient's pain are the same ones arguing that nurses can practice medicine independently of physicians.

In this case, your doctor has written that you are to receive 4 mg of morphine every three hours as needed for pain reported as 7 to 10 in severity. She must give all four milligrams under these orders even if she believes that a lower dose would do.

But things have gotten even more restrictive for her. Your doctor now must also specify the sequence under which she must administer medications, and of course, a physician cannot reasonably write a series of prospective pain medication orders where the milder, oral medication is not tried first. True to form, in your case, your physician has written for you to have two tablets of 5 mg Percocet tablets every three hours for pain in the case of 7 to 10 pain, and he has specified that she must administer the Percocet *before* trying the morphine.

So, off to the medication drawer your nurse goes to get the Percocet knowing full well that the Percocet is not going to cut it. She cannot bypass the Percocet under these circumstances because the software electronically blocks her access to the morphine medication until after she documents having administered Percocet as directed in the orders and has at least opened the drawer in the medicine dispenser housing the Percocet, something for which she would criminally liable if she were to fraudulently do.

Moments later, your nurse returns holding with a cup of water and the two Percocet tablets she is required to give you before she can truly manage your pain. You take the cup with which you are to wash down the medication, spilling some of it because your hands are trembling from the pain. You swallow the medication and wait. For thirty minutes, you lie in your bed careful not to move because it hurts so badly. You call for the nurse to tell her that it still hurts, but she explains to you that she cannot give you the morphine yet because the machine has locked for an hour until you are eligible for morphine.[xiii]

Thirty minutes later, she walks back into the room and asks you to answer a question to which she already knows the answer. "How bad is your pain?"

"Ten, damn it!" you yell, your patience exhausted.

She smiles and walks out of the room and comes back with a syringe full of morphine, which she infuses into your IV. Moments later, you start to feel the relief. Of course, now you have two medications in your system when you could have had only one, and you have unnecessarily spent a little over an hour in pain due to the government's regulatory hand. But you are nevertheless grateful, and you look up at the nurse and thank her.

This regulatorily created dance of inefficiency and goal achievement impediments by no means represents an exception to the interference of how medicine is practiced in medicine. Everything from the perioperative antibiotics you receive to the devices authorized to shave your hair before surgery as been touched by the government through its oversight capacity. Remember that in Chapter 3 we came across the opening statement in the Medicare Act, "Nothing in this subchapter shall be construed to authorize any Federal office or employee to exercise any supervision or control over the practice of medicine or how medical services are provided, or over the selection, tenure, or compensation of any officer or employee of any institution, agency, or person providing health services; or to exercises any supervision or control over the administration or operation of any such institution, agency, or

---

[xiii] Medial dispensers do have override capabilities, but employing them requires verification and supportive explanations. Excessive use of these bypass modalities may be cause for concern for reviewers.

person."[221] At this point, the government is so far past compliance with this mandate, it is as if it were non-existent. Yet somehow, we believe it appropriate to give this same entity even more control over our healthcare. The contention that government would demonstrate self-restraint in a scenario where it controls all of healthcare and that its interventions would be conducive to better healthcare defies reality.

Certificates of Need

Another example of hospital overregulation is certificate of need (CON) legislation. Hospitals were once dependent on their staff physicians to bring them business. It all came down to the hospital's reputation. If a hospital delivered great care to its infirmed and supported their doctors in delivering the highest quality of care, its reputation would flourish and its numbers would surge. If it did not, patients and physicians alike would take their business elsewhere, and the hospital's administrators would quickly recognize they had a problem to fix.

All of this changed with the passage of CON laws. The certificate of need is a government's assertion of the existence of a need to build a hospital within a certain community. Without such a certificate, an investor hoping to build a hospital is unable to do so regardless of the perceived favorability of market conditions. Once the government determines the need for hospitals are met within a community, no further CONs are granted, and the incumbent hospital owns a regional monopoly over the market.

Prior to 1974, CONs as conditions for building hospitals were virtually unknown as these certificates resulted from the passage of the Health Planning Resources Development Act requiring states to enact such laws if they were to maintain their eligibility for certain federal healthcare funding programs. Within four years of the passage of the Act, 36 states passed CON laws, and eventually, 49 out of 50 states enacted them.[222]

The logic of CON legislation flew in the face of every principle of supply and demand. As the reasoning went, hospitals were charging so much for care because there was an oversupply of beds. To pay for the maintenance of these empty beds, hospitals had to overcharge patients inhabiting the beds that were actually being used. However, if the government were to limit the number of hospital beds in a community, then it would counteract the empty bed strain on hospitals, placing them in a position to lower their prices.[223] Additionally, the greater profits amassed by these hospitals would allow them to redirect their capital to the care of the indigent and the needy.[224]

After forty years of CON legislation, prices have predictably risen greatly and here has been no rush of "excess profits" into the community.

As hospitals gained the right to control a region's market, they scurried to establish networks of physicians who worked exclusively for them. These doctors were either employed by the hospital or by a subsidiary of the hospital. A guaranteed flow of patients having been secured, the pressure on hospitals to please their customers and maintain impeccable customer service became less intense. Physicians were considered replaceable and were no longer the principal architects of patient care and quality standards. For the patient, the change often resulted in him or her no longer having a relationship with a physician who owned or worked for a freestanding medical office. Thus, the intimate relationship he or she had with an individual physician was replaced with an impersonal, business relationship with a company.

Macroeconomically, hospitals have become regional oligopolies where they dictate the delivery of care in their communities. Corporate guidelines regarding referral patterns and patient care practices have become the norm. Organizations devoted to the post-hospitalization care of patients now have to kowtow to the hospital and its whims.

In the meantime, between 2007 and 2014 hospital prices rose by 42% (compared to 18% for physician prices) and now account for about 33% of the nation's total healthcare expenditures.[225] And, by the way, there is also no "compelling evidence; that CON laws improved quality or access."[226]

The CON experiment ended in failure, and the Health Planning Resources Act was repealed in 1987, but the damage was done. Even though the federal requirement that states enact CON laws was no longer in place, states did not rush to repeal them. Hospitals with CONs had become deeply entrenched in their communities, employing every legal recourse at their disposal to ward off potential competitors, including the repeal of their state's CON laws. By 2019, only 13 states had discontinued their CON programs.[xiv, 227] In the meantime, hospital prices continue to spike, and networks continue to dictate the terms of care for their subsidiaries and their communities.

The damage from these ill-founded CON laws has clearly not ended.

[xiv] These thirteen states include the twelve states cited in the article by the National Conference of State Legislatures plus Florida, which repealed its program in the 2019 legislative session.

Bundled Payment Models

Another method through which government has sought to manipulate healthcare is through the use of bundled payments. When payments are "bundled," one provider, oftentimes the hospital, is paid an amount of money that covers the hospitalization plus the costs of all expected services for a time following the hospitalization. So, for example, in the case of the hip replacement of which we previously spoke, the hospital would get paid for the cost of the hip replacement, the expected hospitalization, the surgeon, physical therapy, nursing home care, and home health services, among other charges. The hospital then networks with members of each of those sectors, paying them from the money allotted by the payer.

The logic of this payment model is that by placing someone in charge of the cost and coordination of each patient's care, that entity will then work zealously to keep the costs of all the combined services down, as those costs will eat away at the profits that the responsible entity will make from the case. The danger of such a payment model is that it places control for all downstream care in the hands of the bundler, in this case the hospital, whose interests do not always align with those of the patient. Because the amount paid to the bundler (the hospital) is preset, it is pressured into cutting costs at all portions of the patient's care. Thus the hospital will influence the therapist to cut visits and apply pressure to the rehabilitation center physician to shorten the patients' stays. The bundler controls everything, and everyone is dependent on the bundler.

The hospital bundler is also incentivized to open downstream care facilities in the interest of saving money and exercising greater control of the care delivered. It may open its own outpatient physical therapy facilities within a community, forcing the independents out of business. It may also open its own nursing home, outpatient-imaging facilities, and hire its own surgeons.

Such cost savings do not come without a price, and in this case, they are the loss of diversity within a community's healthcare system, a reduction in healthcare options for the patient, and less competition. Through government enacted bundled payment models providers are forced to jump through hoops to accommodate the hospital's needs and interests while bypassing those of the patient. Once again, control of the patient's care is taken away from him and placed at the hands of another. Even more offensive, these transitions in reimbursements are not organically arising in response to demands from a free and efficient market, but from the artificial pricing pressures enacted by government.

Disparities in Reimbursement

At 32% of the nation's health expenditures, by far the largest chunk of our healthcare dollars is devoted to hospital care. This compares to nursing care facilities at 4.8%, physician and clinical services at 19.9%, and prescription drugs at 9%.[228] One would think that policymakers working to artificially cut healthcare costs would target hospital reimbursements. Yet, under Medicare rules, hospital-based services get paid up to ten times more for a procedure performed in a hospital than the identical procedure performed somewhere else. Cardiac catheterizations, for example, are paid at much higher rates when performed in a hospital compared to the same procedure undertaken in a freestanding facility. Providers, therefore, gravitate to hospitals, which outcompete ambulatory surgery centers for reasons having nothing to do with efficiency, quality of care, or cost savings. Not only do these artificial elevations increase the price of the care delivered in hospitals and the percentage of the GDP expended on healthcare, but also they tend to keep innovators from exploring less expensive alternatives to hospitalization for the delivery of identical care.

Hospitals argue these price disparities are needed to accommodate for the higher costs of healthcare delivery in their setting, but generally, they are using their excess gains to hire more physicians, even in specialties outside of those traditionally providing hospital-based services.[229] These physicians are added to massive, hospital-owned networks that drive the smaller, physician-owned private practices out of business and propagate their leverage for maintaining their artificial price elevations. CMS estimates that the disparity for hospital reimbursement in only a few targeted procedures costs Medicare $610 million and their beneficiaries $150 million in extra copays.[230]

Accountable Care Organizations

The appearance of accountable care organizations, or ACOs, is purely the result of government's manipulation of healthcare. These healthcare networks are made up of groups of multispecialty physicians and ancillary healthcare providers who bill for services as a unit. These often-massive groups of providers work in concert to deliver care to their patients from a wide spectrum of specialties and services. When a patient sees her primary doctor for a leg ulcer brought on because of poor circulation, the primary doctor, a member of the ACO, will send the patient to the ACO's vascular surgeon. If the ACO's vascular surgeon needs an ultrasound to assess the integrity of the patient's blood flow to her leg, he sends her to the ACOs radiologist. And when the patient and her doctor agree to undergo surgery, the ACO's vascular surgeon books the case at the hospital belonging to the ACO. Together, they bill for the care of the patient under one administrative roof, sharing its costs and profits.

There are several, very threatening problems with this scheme. Once again, there is an umbrella organization placing pressure on each of its members to not necessarily do what is in the best interests of the patient, but to cut costs wherever it can. The cost-cutting efforts are not just those affecting an individual provider, but the whole group, depersonalizing their decisions and allowing the patient's interests to get lost in the shuffle. Unlike the old health maintenance organization or HMO, the ACO is not a closed system where the patient is not allowed to seek care outside of the insurance created network. Rather, ACOs are open systems where its provider members are strongly incentivized to keep care within their network. Thus, if our patient engages with her primary care provider, the doctor will not refer her to the best surgeon or the one with the most experience in her particular condition, as he could, due to the strong incentive to keep her within the ACO. Of course, hospitals have been very keen in forming their own ACOs, often being the only ones in a community with the resources and capital to do so. Their efforts at creating ACOs that the own help to further consolidate the markets around them while, once again, artificially driving private practices out of business.

Another very disconcerting aspect of ACOs is that their ownership is not limited to healthcare providers or even healthcare centered companies. Any organization, Wal-Mart, Target, Exxon, or General Electric, for example, may get into the business, but not necessarily in the hopes of providing care for its employees as is seen in many ERISA regulated healthcare plans, but merely for the sake of making money in the healthcare industry, but without the associated ingrained interest in caring for others.

Then there are the quality targets imposed upon ACOs in order to maintain full reimbursement for their services,[231] performance objectives and measures implemented by the federal government to satisfy its goals. The reality is that ACOs as a whole have not resulted in a clear improvement in the quality of healthcare. As of this writing, there is no conclusive evidence that the presence of ACOs led to an elevation in the quality of the healthcare delivered. In fact, at least one study has found no difference between the mortality rates amongst hospitalized ACO patients and non-ACO patients.[232]

The ACO is only designed to incentivize cost-cutting with little consideration for the patient, her needs, or her desires. Hospitals and large corporations, in the meantime, continue to profit while increasing their control over the healthcare delivery system, all with the backing of government. Let us recall that the market did not direct for the ACO's appearance. Rather, it was legislatively instituted through payment incentives implemented under the Affordable Care Act.[233]

All these observations lead to the same irrefutable conclusion: healthcare is way too complex, integrated, and intimate to allow one agency or expert to decide the most appropriate directions to be pursued. We have already recognized the most effective entity at identifying a) the best prices; b) the most appropriate quality oversight; and c) the best organizational systems for product delivery. That entity, of course, is the consumer. This is because the consumer is not a single player. Rather, the consumer represents the collective intervention of all participants in a marketplace. Given sufficient time, and sometimes only a very brief period of time, the consumer will always arrive at the correct answer because he or she is engaged in a constant state of trial and error, judging what works and what doesn't. Through the consumer's continuous expressions of his or her preferences by way of his or her wallet there exists a perpetual compass directing the supplier to the best answer, not the perfect one, but the best one. And this is what is needed in healthcare.

Yes, healthcare needs to be regulated and overseen, but it ought not be directed. Instead of aiming at constructing the ideal healthcare delivery system through regulatory oversight, policymakers ought to place the consumer in a better position to pressure the market into delivering the care it demands. When it comes to hospitals and regional healthcare delivery models, the answer is to get out of the way. Let people who are called to care for others dream, develop, and compete, even if for the sake of profit, so long as their passion for caring for their brethren serves as their top priority. For if they can forge a new, virgin path, they will be quickly joined by others eager to deliver their product with similar innovations and even better results at lower prices, beseeching the approval of the ever-wise consumer.

In the world of healthcare delivery, this sage concept translates to allowing hospitals to compete without impediment against each other. Let providers compete against themselves. And let suppliers and manufacturers compete in their arena. So long as the consumer reigns supreme, the manufacturers and providers will not overcharge. They will either have to improve their products or services to gain the consumer's trust, find a way to deliver their products for a better price or step aside to make room for those whose models work better.

If ACOs need exist, let them appear organically, not by fiat. If networks need appear to share their profits and their cost savings, then they will be easily identified by the ever-seeking consumer cognizant of the funds available to spend on their care and demanding that the best prices be offered for the privilege of their business. If the suppliers can truly improve quality, let them do so through their own innovations. The consumer will quickly identify who is providing the better products or services and who is not.

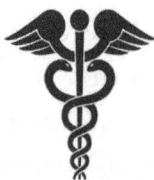

Chapter 4

The Cost of Socialized Medicine

In socialism, government owns the means of production and controls the distribution of society's assets. Its advocates claim that under such a system, each member will be tasked with supplying only what he can and will be provided with what he needs. "From each according to his ability, to each according to his needs."[234] Applied to healthcare, socialists claim that under their system people would no longer have to worry about receiving the healthcare they need. Such services would be available to all since there would be no uninsured.

American socialists feign dismay as they lament at how the United States of America, the single wealthiest nation in the world, does not provide "free" healthcare for all. If the United States would only adopt the socialistic principles of common ownership and utilitarian distribution, they claim, it would possess the greatest healthcare delivery system on earth, not the paltry, corrupt, and ineffective system in place today.

From the time of Adam Smith and *The Wealth of Nations*, economists have recognized the most cost-efficient, most inclusive system for the delivery of products or services, is the free market. Like a living organism searching for the most efficient method of supporting itself, the free market is continuously working on developing the least tasking methods of conjuring, producing, transporting, and exchanging goods and services. Any regulation interfering with its natural, resting steady state represents a corruption of this most precise, lean process and a strain on its economy.

What's more, even if government tried to undertake such massive investments in researching market efficiencies, it still would not be able to arrive at the innovations of the free market because each "expert" would never be as motivated and dedicated to finding that one advantage in production and delivery as could the person whose very livelihood depends on profiting from the improvement. In fact, too many improvements can only be identified through living the process, something that government experts never do.

If there is one thing we have recurrently seen, it is that when government or regulators intervene in the natural workings of the free market, they make the system less efficient, less streamlined, and often, more dangerous. This is certainly true with healthcare. There is a cost to government-run healthcare that most analysts view only in terms of pecuniary considerations. We will not repeat that mistake here, for although there is a monetary price to be paid for government-run healthcare, there is one intangible cost that supersedes any financial consideration of such a system: the loss of the patient's autonomy.

The Intangible Costs of Government-Run Healthcare

Allowing a government to make decisions regarding the most intimate parts of a person's existence is so threatening that it ought to be completely eliminated from consideration, especially in a country built under the assumption that its government should honor the supremacy of the people. In the United States, governmental authority is said to emanate from the people. If government were placed in a position to control and administer the healthcare of the people who gave it its powers, the foundational relationship between man and government would be flipped on its head. Given the authority to administer the nation's healthcare, government would decide what healthcare goods and services are appropriate for its population. It alone would determine what services warrant purchasing and distribution to its population and which do not. In effect, government would be empowered with deciding who gets to live and who gets to die. Therefore, the citizen, the analysis is on handing healthcare to the government is quite simple. Either the government can dictate the availability of life-preserving and life-extending procedures and make the people subservient to it, or it does not, and government continues to be subservient to the people. Only one of the two situations is possible, not both.

A single-payer healthcare system would be the death knell of the patient-physician relationship because the physician, whether employed by the government or "independently operating," would be in no position to autonomously design the best treatment for his or her patient. The doctor's allegiance would necessarily lie with the entity regulating the profession and not with the patient. Innovation, too, would be hit, as there would be no demand for any product except through the approval and consent of government. No longer would inventors and manufacturers be sniffing out opportunities through the identification of new markets demanded by the people. Instead, they would be conspiring to learn what the government wished to see come to fruition and guess the needs of the healthcare industry as identified by the government. In such a monopsony, what would be better than to bribe, pressure, and cajole the single purchaser of products into demanding your goods or services to the exclusion of all others?

And then there are the government-mandated health optimization efforts. Are you fat? Obesity costs money and since the government is responsible for saving as much money as possible, it can mandate that you not be obese, or at the very least prohibit items from reaching you that cause obesity. If government is in charge of who gets healthcare, then you can be made ineligible to receive benefits until you lose weight, cap your fat intake, or exercise a certain minimum amount. And if you believe this possibility is too far fetched to happen in the United States, recall that New York banned 32-ounce soft drinks, and public schools throughout the nation were impeded from serving offensive foods such as pizza all in the name of combating obesity. Additionally, the FDA banned trans-fats from the American "food supply" stating they are no longer "Generally Recognized as Safe"[235] even though they were never recognized as being a principal cause of heart disease. In the meantime tobacco products, which are the single most important cause of lung cancer and directly responsible for millions of deaths in the United States, are not banned. Why should 32-ounce sodas, which have never caused anyone's death nor identified as a principal cause of obesity, be banned while tobacco products are not? Such is the arbitrary and capricious nature of government and its regulations.

In other countries where socialized medicine prevails, intrusions on personal liberties in the name of healthcare have been implemented in forms much more prevalent than those encountered in the United States. In England, smokers were banned from undergoing elective surgical procedures.[236, 237] And in some areas of the country, obese patients are not offered surgery until they attain a body mass index of less than 30, not because the surgery is unduly risky, but simply to save money.[xv, 238] This is what can be expected if government is given the authority to supervise the public's healthcare system. Why? Because government must contain costs in administering a nation's healthcare, and it can reasonably argue that to do so, it must take these necessary measures restricting lifestyles or punishing noncompliance. Oh, and by the way, it's good for you.

In short, the cost of socialized medicine will exceed most objectively predicted consequences. It will be disastrous in a manner much grander than finances and money. The adoption of socialized medicine represents a serious if not mortal blow to the concept of personal independence and to the idea that patients ought to be free to decide what is best for them without intrusion from the government of external entities.

That's not to say that the financial implications of adopting a government-run, universal healthcare scheme wouldn't be devastating as well. They will, a consideration we take up next.

Funding a Single-Payer Healthcare System

From a financial perspective, the primary consideration behind the Left's interest in promoting a single-payer system is reducing the nation's healthcare expenditures. They contend that Americans spend too much on healthcare, so much so that it is causing a drag on the nation's economy. The amount of money being spent on healthcare is consuming the nation's wealth and keeping it from realizing its full potential. As the advocates describe it, America is spending approximately 17.9% of its GDP on healthcare alone;[239]

[xv] To give you a sense of what a BMI of 30 is like, a 6'1" and 230 lbs. person has a BMI of 31. A 5'8" person weighing 143 lbs. has a BMI of 30.

a number far exceeding that spent by any other developed country. Therefore, they argue, it is incumbent upon us to reform the system to curtail these excess expenditures.

But for the Left, of course, the responsibility of improving this situation falls squarely upon government. If the problem finds that too much of the nation's money is devoted to healthcare, then the solution is to have government cut the nation's healthcare expenditures. Advocates contend that single-payer or government-run system of healthcare delivery can easily accomplish this goal through reductions in administrative expenses and by cutting reimbursement to healthcare providers and drug manufacturers.[xvi]

According to the advocates for centralized healthcare, if their plans are not adopted, the cost of healthcare over the next ten years will be $32 trillion. But this figure only accounts for the cost to the federal government and does not represent the total costs to the nation, a figure known as national health expenditure (NHE),[240] which includes those amounts spent by government, third party payees, and individuals. If reformers are truly concerned about the percentage of the GDP spent on healthcare, it is actually the NHE they should want to cut.

But the actual numbers regarding the beneficial effects of their proposed changes do not support their contentions. According to estimates by Charles Blahous through the Mercatus Center and George Washington University, if there was no reform, the nation would spend approximately $50.271 trillion over ten years on healthcare.[241] Under a single-payer plan, the costs would be $48.834 trillion, but only if there is an associated 40% decrease in provider reimbursement.[242] The difference between doing nothing and adopting

---

[xvi] Even though, as we saw earlier, physician and clinical services account for only 19.9% of the nation's healthcare expenditures and prescription drugs for 9%.

a single-payer healthcare system, *in light of a 40% decrease in provider reimbursement,* is a mere $1.437 trillion over ten years, or 3%![243]

Yet, from our prior analyses, we know how unlikely it is that a 40% cut in provider reimbursement will be realized and how threatening such a cut would be to patients through the loss of providers and the diminution of quality candidate recruitment. As evidenced by the Medicaid experience, a 40% reduction in provider reimbursement will result in a dramatic egress of physicians from the market and their eventual substitution with much lower quality and likely fewer doctors. Patients will be intensely dissatisfied with the system, and perhaps even witness its near collapse. The contention that the nation's healthcare delivery system would continue to function under the strain of a 40% cut in reimbursement is simply not credible.

On the other hand, if we assume that no cuts in reimbursement were to be realized, the projected national healthcare expenditure over ten years would be $53.086 trillion, an *increase* of 2.815 trillion, or 5%![244] Regardless of a 40% cut or not, the increase in government spending on healthcare will be $32.1 trillion over ten years!

Therefore, according to our best predictions on a very unpredictable topic, what will change if a Medicare-For-All styled reform for healthcare delivery is adopted is not the total amount we spend on healthcare. That will remain the same at about $50 trillion give or take 5%. What will change is the source of the funding, from primarily private sources to overwhelming government funding. And along with that, there will follow a migration of authority from the individual to the unelected, virtually invisible bureaucrat.

What's more, as the expenditure numbers climb, government will respond in a historically predictable and reproducible way: rationing. Government has too because unless it rations care, the percentage of GDP that will be expended on healthcare will remain unchanged, which is unacceptable to those who implemented the system in the first place.

So really the whole debate over how to fund the nation's health-care system comes down to one question: should we sign up for a massive increase in our tax liability to purchase a system of health-care delivery over which we will have very little say and no chance of curbing the healthcare expenditures, or should we keep health-care safely in our hands?

There is also the issue of how such a large increase in gov-ernment spending would be funded. There are only seven ways through which healthcare can be funded: premiums, cost-sharing, taxes, personally financed healthcare, institutional expenditures, charitable contributions, and borrowing. Of these, only two of them: premiums, cost-sharing, taxes, and borrowing are available to the government. The last of these, borrowing, is illusory since the government would really not be paying for anything through borrowing, but rather merely delay its payment.

It is therefore likely that if Congress were to proceed with a mandatory, single-payer, national insurance program, it would do so through higher taxes for revenue collection and allocating those funds to the nation's healthcare insurance network.[xvii]

And how much would our taxes need to be increased? Enough to fund another $32.1 trillion over ten years or $12,637.80 for every adult American per year.[xviii] If the government were to take

[xvii] Note that no matter what a law may look like when it is first passed, a pres-ent Congress cannot bind a future Congress, allowing the law to be changed. In considering the propriety of passing such a massive tax, we must keep in mind that Congress has repeatedly demonstrated a pattern of obfuscating such funds and using them for other purposes. Such was the case with Social Security and Medicare, both of which presently run the risk of bankruptcy due, at least in part, to the practice of using the funds collected from the people to finance other government programs.

[xviii] $32.1 trillion ÷10 years ÷ 254 million estimated adult Americans= $12,637.80.

over the totality of the nation's healthcare costs, the goal expressed by single-payer advocates, it would need to raise enough money to pay for the projected NHE over ten years, or approximately $50 trillion. The tax bill for healthcare to cover the NHE with a 40% reduction in provider reimbursement (which is unlikely to be achieved) would be $19,225.98 per year.[xix] Without the 40% provider reimbursement cuts, the healthcare tax bill for each American adult would be $20,900 per year![xx]

To be clear, this would be the tax bill imposed on every adult American, regardless of his or her ability to pay, and would only cover the healthcare portion of the nation's budget. Americans would still have to pay for the national defense, social security, roads, infrastructure, etc., with money that goes beyond this exorbitant bill. Of course, every American adult cannot pay over $19,000, or even $12,000, per year to the federal government. So, who would?

Well, if we impose the bill on the top 1% of income earners, as some advocating for a single-payer healthcare propose, then the bill on those top 1% income earners would range from $2,090,000 and $1,263,789,000 per year, an impossible amount since the average yearly income for the nation's top 1% of income earners is $1.32 million per year.[245]

Alternatively, some proponents, such as Senator Elizabeth Warren, suggest charging the nation's billionaires for the nation's healthcare bill. But here again, we run into problems since the total wealth of all American billionaires *combined* is only about $3.363 trillion.[xxi] So, even if the proponents were sufficiently brazen to steal all the

[xix] $48.834 trillion ÷10 years ÷ 254 million estimated adult Americans =$19,225.98.

[xx] $53.086 trillion ÷10 years ÷ 254 million estimated adult Americans=$20,900.00.

[xxi] This estimate is obtained by adding up the combined estimated wealth of all American billionaires in the 2019 Forbes 400 list and the Bloomberg Billionaires Index.

American billionaires' wealth, the stash would only pay for about one year of the single-payer reform plan.

Senator Bernie Sanders proposes a hybrid system of raising revenue. First, he would implement a 7.5% income-based premium upon employers, raising $3.9 trillion over ten years. A 4% premium would be charged on all American households, which would raise an additional $3.5 trillion over ten years. He would then charge the "rich" more in taxes raising another $1.8 trillion over ten years. The estate tax would be raised by another $249 billion and a wealth tax on the top 0.1 would raise another $1.3 trillion. Closing the Gingrich-Edwards Loophole[xxii] for wealthy business owners would raise another $247 billion, and a one-time fee of $767 billion over ten years would be imposed on corporate offshore profits. Large financial institutions would be required to pay over $117 billion over ten years and the elimination of a commonly employed accounting trick would help raise another $112 billion over ten years.[246]

Without subtracting any negative effects Senator Sanders' proposal would have on the American economy, his fund generating program would raise a mere $11.55 trillion, far short of the $32.1 trillion in tax increases required to fund the Medicare-For-All program and even further from the $48 trillion to $53 trillion required to fully take on the country's national health expenditure. In fact, the amount Senator Sanders predicts could be raised through his fundraising efforts isn't even enough to fund his woefully under-predicted cost increase of $13.8 trillion.

[xxii] The Gingrich-Edwards Loophole is a condition within the law that allows owners of S-corporations to avoid paying money into Medicare and Social Security. Mark Koba, "How the Gingrich Edwards-Tax Loophole Works, CNBC (blog), March 5, 2014, accessed on Jan. 22, 2020, https://www.cnbc.com/2014/03/05/cnbc-explains-the-gingrich-edwards-tax-loophole.html; "TAX GAP Actions Needed to Address noncompliance with S Corporation Tax Rules," Report to the Committee on Finance, U.S. Senate, GAO, December 2009, https://www.gao.gov/new.items/d10195.pdf.

As we can see, no proposal would allow government to fund the nation's healthcare bills without exorbitant cuts in the healthcare products and services available to Americans; i.e. rationing. Fortunately, there is another, more effective way of achieving a superior healthcare system for a lower cost while retaining our foundational integrity and our autonomy. Such a solution lies with the free market.

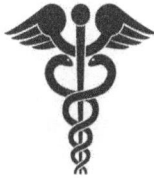

Julio Gonzalez

Chapter 5

Challenges to Healthcare Delivery

Throughout the twentieth century and into the twenty-first, policymakers have focused on government as the primary tool with which to address issues regarding healthcare delivery. Not only does this approach run counter to the principles inherent to the nation's foundation, but it has tended to suppress the industry, strip it of its flexibility, and encumber the opportunities for organic solution implementation. Either through ignorance, habit, or lack of resolve, many refuse to give the matter a fresh look and even more are hesitant to offer solutions to the problems that confront us that don't increase the ambit of government. But if government has been the catalyst of increasing difficulties, then perhaps more effective solutions lie elsewhere. Here, we address some of our present healthcare challenges.

The Erosion of the Patient-Physician Relationship

Our interactions with our doctors are amongst the most intimate, private, and confidential exchanges we experience. What's more, the recipient of the information is expected to be completely loyal to us, not only in safeguarding the information he or she has gained, but in employing it in the most judicious manner possible.

What's more, once the physician constructs the best answer for our ailment, we expect him or her to be able to implement the plan without obstruction or interference.

Tragically, this is not what takes place in our country.

The issue of confidentiality of medical information is no longer a simple matter of the physician keeping his or her mouth shut and storing our medical records in a secure space within his or her office. Presently, the overwhelming number of physicians keeps some form of electronic medical records. This change towards electronic medical records was largely dictated through the passage of the American Recovery and Reinvestment Act of 2009 where participants in Medicare were required to demonstrate the "meaningful use" of electronic medical records or face penalties.

The transition, of course, was not driven by consumer demand nor by the greater economic efficiency adoption of digital records would allow. Just the opposite is true. The implementation of electronic medical records has been an expensive undertaking that government incentives only partially offset.[247] Estimates for the cost of merely implementing electronic medical records run from $26,000.00 to $43,000.00 per physician. And the adoption of these records foreseeably caused significant problems relating to the privacy of patient interactions with their physicians.

In 2015, for example, Medical Informatics Engineering, Inc., an electronic medical records company, had private information on approximately 3.5 million people stolen from its servers,[248] and in 2018, a Michigan based company reported a breach of 15,027 patient records.[249] The problem has grown to such an extent that in April 2019 alone, the number of organizations reporting data breaches reached a record high of 44 with a total of 963,794 compromised medical records.[250] *In one month!*

But it isn't just the hackers that pose privacy threats. The sale of patient information has also become problematic. Amazingly, the courts have ruled that the sale of patient-specific data by pharmacies with data mining companies is a constitutionally protected act.[251] Additionally, hospitals have been required to share patient information with state data services. This data then becomes publicly available through public disclosure laws. So specific is the information provided to these state agencies that it may be used to target specific individuals, either through human or automated methods. [252]

But it's not just the data mining and hacking that make one's records less than private, a patient's third-party payer has a right to directly access its client's records, and in some cases, so do the state and federal governments. The concern over the ultimate destinations of one's medical information and its collateral use prompted gun rights groups in Florida to attempt to prohibit physicians from inquiring about the presence of guns in a home during routine office visits for fear that such information would end up in some government database. Although passed, that legislation was ultimately overturned in federal court. The issue of government accessing non-medical information contained within a patient's medical records still stands unaddressed.[253]

Separate from the external influence of third-party payers is a physician's employer. Here again, government meddling has propped up the threat, and it all relates to liberal policymakers' obsession with promoting the development of large healthcare networks. If physicians from multiple specialties could organize under one roof, the proponents of centralized control of healthcare conclude, then patients would be more able to seamlessly and less expensively move throughout the medical specialties with less room for medical errors. But by imposing these herculean organizational structures upon the public, the physician's loyalty is moved away from his or her patient. Rather, it is shared with his or her allegiance to the organization employing him or her and with the policy directives designed to earn his employer its bonus; a bonus earned through compliance with directives ultimately created by the federal government.

The result of these intrusions is palpable. Increasingly, physicians are beholden to something other than their patients. In 2016, for the first time in American history, less than 50% of physicians (47.1%) owned their practices, compared to 76.1% in 1983 and 53.2% in 2012.[254]

Additionally, the physician is striving to see more patients in less time. Due to the increasing time constraints placed on doctors, patients call their interactions less satisfying and incomplete. They report feeling like mere numbers in a giant system where individual needs don't really matter. Those impressions are heightened by the controlling entity's willingness to exchange one doctor for another in treating its clients. Physicians are no longer free to construct and implement the best plans for their patients without external interference. And although the statisticians and the epidemiologists may be happy because the appropriate boxes are being checked, the patients are not.[255, 256]

All these issues amount to a massive and unrelenting erosion of the primacy of the patient-physician relationship, the most important pillar in any healthcare system. If a patient cannot trust that her personal information will be held confidentially, if she cannot feel confident that the doctor's allegiance is primarily to her, or if she believes that powers beyond her control are determining whether she can obtain the best possible care or not, then American healthcare is merely a shell of a system propped up by the massive volumes of paper and regulations. Once we lose this central pillar to healthcare delivery and human decency, further attempts at solving problems in healthcare are futile.

A healthcare delivery system based on the free market will go a long way towards solving these problems if for no other reason than it places the patient in control of the care he or she receives and the decisions being made on his or her behalf. By definition, the patient will once again feel like the physician is there for him or her. Patient confidentiality will be bolstered because the physician's allegiance will not be diluted by either a third-party payer or by government. And if patients demand that their doctors be members of either a solo practice or a small group of like-minded physicians, then that model will win out through the vote of the wallet. In short, a free market healthcare delivery system will protect the most important facet of healthcare, the sanctity of the patient-physician relationship because such a system necessarily makes the doctor beholden to only one person: the patient.

The Cost of Accessing Care

The supposedly high cost of healthcare is the most frequently cited complaint from healthcare care reform advocates. As noted in Chapter 4, in 2017, Americans spent $3.2 trillion on healthcare or 17.9% of the gross domestic product. According to. the noted healthcare policy pundit and advocate for centralized healthcare, Dr. Ezekiel Emanuel, "Higher costs mean families decide coverage is too expensive. State budgets are strained, leading to higher Medicaid costs and higher premiums for state employees. Ultimately, the high costs accelerate the shrinking of the middle class,...affects our standing, [and]...undermines our abilities to do things."[257]

Of the total amounts spent on healthcare, hospital care amounted to $1.1 trillion, physician reimbursement and clinical services
took up $694 billion, prescription drugs was $333.4 billion, resi-
dential and personal services took up $183.1 billion, nursing care
facilities accounted for $166.3 billion, dental services $129.1 billion, and other services such as durable medical equipment, nondu-
rable medical equipment, and other professional services made up
3% of the remainder or less.[258] As far as funding is concerned, $1.2
trillion (34%) came from private insurance, $705.9 billion (20%)
from Medicare, and Medicaid paid for $581.9 billion (17%). Only
10% of healthcare funding, or $365.5 billion, was realized through
personal funds.[259]

But what if 17.9% of the GDP is what Americans want to
spend on their healthcare? Don't Americans have the right to spend
as much as they want on a certain product or industry?

The fact is that, although many like Dr. Emanuel argue the United States is spending too much on healthcare, no one has determined
the appropriate amount it wants to spend on healthcare because so
much is subsidized by government or nongovernmental entities. In
other words, because the people themselves are not directly expressing the value of the various healthcare goods and services, we have
no idea of how much they would be willing to pay if the costs were
being borne by them directly. In fact, in determining what the appropriate amount the United States should be spending on healthcare
all we have to go by are the economists' views on the matter and
comparisons with the expenditures of other nations whose cultures
and economics are not comparable with those of the United States.[260]

There may be valid reasons why Americans are opting to pay
more for healthcare than other countries. Data produced by the
World Health Organization in 2000 demonstrated a linear correlation

between the responsiveness of a nation's healthcare system and the percentage of the nation's GDP devoted to it.[261] Consequently, what Americans may be paying for is responsiveness. In other words, at least some of the extra healthcare expenditure in the United States is being allocated to ensuring that when patients are sick, truly sick, they have a team of healthcare personnel and their supporting resources readily available. They may be less concerned with the development of a large population health network as they in knowing that there are people ready to treat them when they need to be treated. This is also the reason why foreigners with complicated and demanding conditions come to the United States, the same reason why most people with hopeless medical situations come to the United States for access to the latest and most intricate advances in medicine.

Despite these observations, however, there is no doubt that America's healthcare system could be even better. It could shine brighter and could be much more affordable while keeping the same levels of responsiveness, ingenuity, expertise, and innovation.

For example, one of the places where America's healthcare system is least efficient is at its point of initial access, which too often is the emergency room. Access to the emergency room is protected in the United States under the Emergency Medical Treatment and Labor Act (EMTALA), but the price of care in these facilities can be over ten times higher than the delivery of the same care through a primary care physician.[262] Hospitals and physicians assigned to the emergency room are required to attend to emergency room patients regardless of the patient's acuity or ability to pay until the patient is stabilized. This stopgap measure is what guarantees healthcare access to all in the United States, but it is not the best method for accessing subacute care.

In 2016, there were over 145 million emergency room visits in the United States.[263] Of these, 13%-27% were not emergencies.[264]

If these patients had presented to the appropriate setting about $4.4 billion of healthcare cost savings would have been realized.[265]

Advocates for centralized healthcare posit that people are accessing care in the emergency room rather than in a more appropriate setting because they have no other place to go. But again, the data does not support their contention.

With the passage of the ACA, the number of uninsured in the United States dropped by approximately 20 million people. However, the same year the ACA was implemented, the number of emergency room visits rose to the highest levels ever recorded at 141.4 million visits.[266, 267] This finding is actually worse than the one in the Oregon Experiment, which found no difference between the uninsured and newly insured Medicaid patients regarding access to care, but also identified an associated increase in resource utilization.[268] Further, although being privately insured seems to be associated with a lower mortality rate,[269] increasing insurance coverage rates within a population resulted in a higher number of visits to the emergency room, not a decrease.[270] Thus, the hypothesis that increasing insurance coverage would result in lower costs through improved non-urgent utilization at the expense of emergency room visits seems to be unsubstantiated.

But how about preventive care? Would facilitating patient access to preventive medicine lower healthcare expenditures? Here again, the answer is no. In 2013, the Congressional Budget Office (CBO) undertook a study to determine whether increasing tobacco excise taxes by 50¢ to better fund preventive care programs would result in lower healthcare expenditures. It did not. According to the CBO and as depicted in Figure 5-1, federal revenues did increase due to the excise tax, and it did decrease the deficit, but this was due largely to the increased revenue stream caused by the new tax, not through health improvement.[271] Although the implementation of a $41 billion program designed to reduce healthcare spending initially caused an approximately 0.01% decrease in spending, as the population aged, the trend reversed, resulting in a similar, spending increase.

Figure 5-1: Relationship between Increase Spending on Preventive Care from a Cigarette Excise Tax and Healthcare Spending.

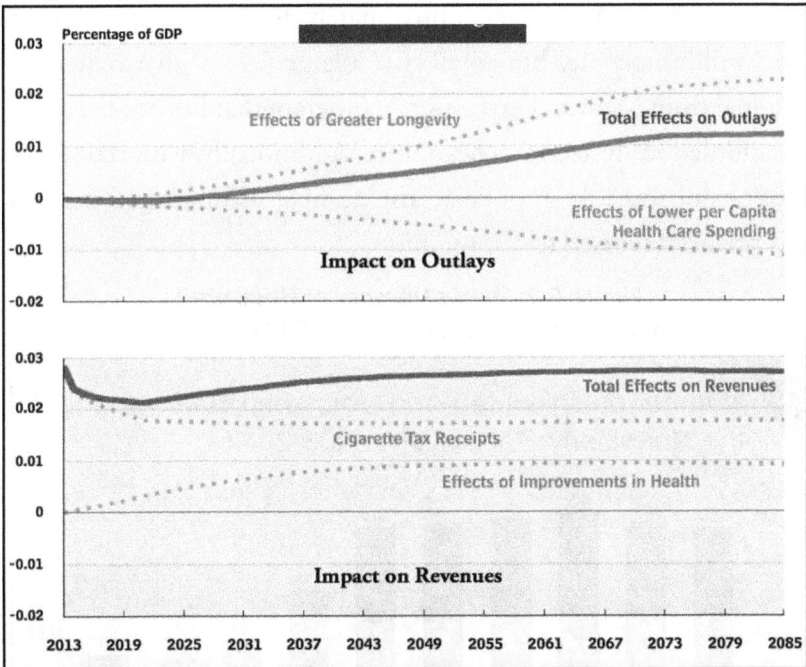

"Raising the Excise Tax on Cigarettes: Effect on Health and the Federal Budget," CBO, Jun. 2012, accessed Jul. 25, 2019, http://www.cbo.gov/sites/default/files/cbofiles/attachments/06-13-Smoking Reduction.pdf.

Additionally, two studies published in Health Affairs shed doubt on the usefulness of organized preventive medicine efforts. One found workplace wellness programs did not bend the cost curve although they shifted the burden from unhealthy employees to healthy one, [272] and another found the coordinated care models supported by accountable care organizations did not lead to cost savings.[273] Even *The New York Times*, an ardent proponent of centralized healthcare, admitted that massive efforts at cost containment through either greater insurance coverage or robust preventive medicine efforts were not associated with significant cost savings.[274]

The persistence of a large uninsured population despite the ACA represents a continuing challenge to America's healthcare system. According to Figure 5-2, the number of uninsured has diminished under the ACA from approximately 44.2 million to a low of 26.7 million people. But recall that a large part of that reduction resulted from Medicaid expansion, a program that has not necessarily afforded ready access to healthcare. Additionally, with the recent erosions of some ACA policies, the number of uninsured persons has predictably risen to 27.4 million.

Figure 5-2: Yearly Number of Uninsured in the United States between 2008 and 2017.

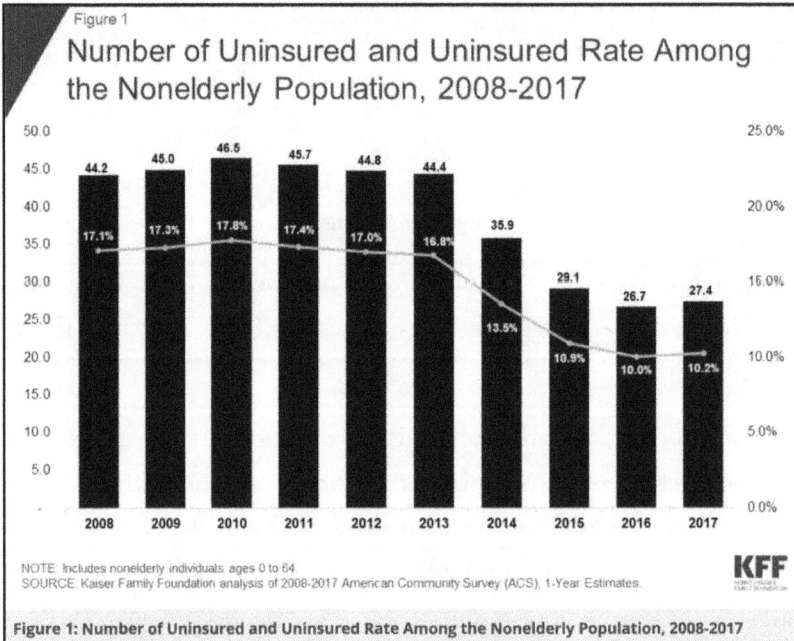

Figure 1: Number of Uninsured and Uninsured Rate Among the Nonelderly Population, 2008-2017

"Key Facts About the Uninsured Population" Kaiser Family Foundation, Dec. 7, 2018, Fig. 1, accessed Jul. 30, 2019, https://www.kff.org/uninsured/fact-sheet/key-facts-about-the-uninsured-population/#.

Although a great deal of time is spent discussing the number of uninsured patients in the United States, the real issue is accessibility. If the whole population was uninsured, but everyone could easily access care when they needed it, there wouldn't be a reason to have a policy discussion regarding the size of the uninsured population. On the other hand, if everyone was covered, but access was atrocious, only the disingenuous would claim that America's healthcare system was exemplary.

So, assuming that those who are insured in our present system have reasonable access to healthcare, why do the uninsured have such difficulty accessing care? A recent Kaiser Family Foundation report offers some key insights into this question.[275] There, 50% of uninsured patients went without care because they did not have a routine place to go. Surprisingly, only 20% of uninsured patients cited cost considerations as their reason for not accessing care with only 24% postponing care because of costs. Relatedly, about the same percentages of uninsured (19%) indicated they either postponed or failed to procure prescription medications due to cost. So, despite our preconceived notions regarding cost being the great motivator for people without insurance to go without care, it seems the lack of an established relationship with a provider is actually the major stumbling block.

From these insights, it is reasonable to conclude that the use of government as the source to solve the challenges associated with funding care and improving its access may not be the correct conduit at all, a conclusion upon which the Framers arrived over two centuries ago, and we seemed to have abandoned.

Pre-existing Conditions

Another issue facing America's healthcare system is the challenge of taking care of people with pre-existing conditions. The issue is somewhat spurious in that it is purely the product of how health-care is funded. We all have conditions. The only thing making them pre-existing is that they were present before a certain event, in this case, the application for insurance coverage. If we were to get rid of the event, namely the application for insurance, then there would be no such thing as a pre-existing condition. They would merely be conditions.

From the insurance company's standpoint, there must be some ability to denote higher-risk patients from others. In the past, the applicant's age, health habits, and number and "pre-existing conditions" played a substantial role in determining whether to cover a new client. Insurers subjected applicants to an underwriting process designed to identify risk factors that could potentially turn that client into a healthcare consumer and that would predict the magnitude of that risk. Treatment for some medical conditions afflicting the applicant would be inexpensive or perhaps not required all. These could be covered through the base premium price. Some conditions could be dealt with by adding an extra charge to the base premium. Others still were deemed so expensive or risky to the insurer that it would refuse to contract with the applicant. People with these conditions would have no ability to obtain coverage from a private payer. Generally, these were people with complicated and involved, chronic medical conditions such as advanced lupus, renal failure, and cancer, among others, and were said to be uninsurable.

There is another group of individuals with "pre-existing conditions." These are people who have developed a condition that was not so expensive or chronic as to place them in the uninsurable category, but who waited until after they developed the medical condition before obtaining insurance. Examples of these conditions include ankle fractures, hypertension, and surgical urgencies.

Insurers protected themselves from these situations by placing a six-month exclusion clause on these "pre-existing conditions." Thus, if one had previously contracted hypertension, insurance companies would not cover its treatment until the beneficiary had signed up with the insurer for a minimum period, say six months. Although this position on the part of insurers was reasonable, the quagmire occurred when someone with hypertension, ulcerative colitis, or diabetes was already covered by a third-party payer and needed to change insurance. This person was then caught in the situation where the condition would not be covered while she put in the necessary time with the new insurer to qualify. The already insured felt like she was stuck with her insurer, and if the product was provided through her employer, she was stuck with her job, too.

Some beneficiaries with employer-based insurance plans were in situations where they could never stop working for fear of losing all coverage. Employer-based plans are group plans, not individual ones. As such insurers would be willing to take on some clients with more involved medical conditions that would have otherwise disqualified the applicant because the employer was bringing a group of enrollees (all of his employees), not just one individual. Here, the insurer would take on the totality of the group's risk making the coverage of certain higher-risk employees with pre-existing conditions manageable. But here again, some were trapped in their jobs knowing that although they may have qualified for participation in the group's plan, they would never qualify for coverage as individuals. They were stuck.

Congress aimed to solve this problem through the passage of the ACA. Under the Act, not only were all employers with greater than 50 employees required to purchase healthcare insurance for their employees (the so-called employer mandate), but Congress dictated the types of plans that were eligible for compliance as well.

For those persons who were either self-employed, or employed by a company with 50 or fewer employees, there was the individual mandate. These people were required, under pain of a tax, to purchase healthcare insurance on their own, and once again Congress defined the minimum criteria the purchase plan would have to meet to qualify.

Concurrently, Congress did away with the whole underwriting process, such that individual and group purchasers alike would no longer have their eligibility or their premiums determined by the extent of their pre-existing conditions or risk factors. In short, the insurer was required to sign up the brittle diabetic as quickly as it would the athlete, and at the same price. As a matter of fact, the only applicant factors an insurer could consider in determining premiums were age and smoking status.[xxiii]

The ACA also set up the incredibly awkward situation where a person could opt out of buying health insurance until after he or she got sick or injured. It was a situation destined for financial failure unless insurance companies were propped up by government subsidies, which is exactly what the ACA did.

As it turned out, the government's model did not work and insurance products slowly but steadily exited the market under the strain of an unfavorable actuarial environment, while premiums, the major target for Obamacare, continued to rise.

[xxiii] I always thought there was a constitutional challenge here for smokers, either through equal protection or due process violations.

Being that the ACA is being eroded through a combination of congressional actions and judicial rulings, the country is still confronted with the question of how to provide healthcare coverage opportunities for those with expensive medical conditions. The exact number of people dealing with this problem is a matter of some controversy, but a 2015 report by the Kaiser Family Foundation gives us a clue. It found a little over 52 million non-elderly people, or 27% of the American, non-elderly population, suffer from at least one condition that would be declinable if insurance companies were allowed to turn applicants away for pre-existing conditions.[276] The HHS also came up with an estimate finding the ratio between uninsurables and insurables to be as high as one in two Americans.[277]

These numbers are indeed startling, but they are likely an overestimation of the magnitude of the problem since they include many who are already obtaining insurance through government-run programs such as Medicare and Medicaid. A better indicator is the number of people who were actually rejected by insurers. A 2010 memorandum from the House Committee on Energy and Commerce reported that the four largest private payers denied coverage to over 651,000 people because of pre-existing conditions between 2007 and 2009.[278] The Committee cautioned the number could be higher since its study did not account for those who were may not have applied for private-payer healthcare coverage due to their medical conditions.[279]

Another measure is the number of persons covered by the Pre-existing Condition Insurance Plan (PCIP), a temporary stop-gap insurance product created under the ACA to temporarily cover those with pre-existing conditions until such time that the underwriting prohibition took effect in 2014. Although expectations were that over 200,000 people would join, by 2012, the number actually participating in the program was a little over 56,000 people.[280] Additionally, there were approximately 220,000 people enrolled at the time in state-run, high-risk pools designed to cover those with pre-existing conditions, for a total of about 260,000 people.[281]

The ACA, the government's approach of ensuring coverage for the uninsured, cost $940 billion over ten years according to President Obama and $1.76 trillion over the same period according to the CBO.[282] Significantly, the Obama estimate does not include the $250 billion needed to correct the outdated and flawed physician reimbursement formula (the SGR) that the Obama Administration cut out of the plan so he could claim the program would cost less than $1 trillion. That reimbursement correction was ultimately implemented in 2015 through the passage of MACRA.[283] More recently the CBO reported that in 2018 the number of subsidies allotted through the ACA would add up to $685 billion with 29 million people still lacking insurance and an estimated 35 million uninsured by 2028.[284]

Despite all of its interventions and costs, the ACA was unable to successfully address the issue of access throughout the wide spectrum of financial and medical circumstances affecting the nation's citizenry. We have already seen how the ACA failed those unable or unwilling to purchase health insurance. Now, we are confronted with the interrelated problem facing those too sick, disabled, or injured to qualify for insurance. For the former, the data strongly suggest that a nongovernmental strategy may be the better answer. For the latter, the best answer would be one where the pre-existence of a condition would not even be a factor in determining access sine the patient's funding source would follow him or her, regardless of employer or location of residence, throughout for life. In Chapter 6, we address how this can be accomplished.

End-of-Life Care

Thus far, we have discussed some of the policy shortcomings associated with a highly regulated healthcare delivery system. We have addressed economic issues, the assault on the patient-physician relationship, and the continued accessibility issues oftentimes exacerbated by government intervention. But arguably the single, biggest threat associated with government intervention in healthcare is its control of access, particularly at the end of one's life.

Approximately 25% of Medicare's budget is spent on an estimated 5% of patients in their last year of life.[285] For some, this category represents a fertile opportunity to cut costs. Viewed in the same light as fraud, waste, and abuse, they categorize these expenditures as wasteful and unnecessary. If only we could cut down on these futile expenditures, they say, government could allocate those funds to people whose lives and productivity could be extended.

All sorts of ideas have been proposed on how government could make these decisions. Yet under each of these, the power of the government stood to be enhanced even to the point that no one, not even the self-paying individual, would be allowed to pay for continued life-saving efforts once the experts determined their futility. Essentially, once the physician determined that life-extending interventions were futile, only palliative care would be available to the patient.

In my first healthcare policy book, *Health Care Reform: The Truth*, I argued against these ideas by stating that there may be a point beyond which access to public funds could be halted, and as opposed to the proposals I was countering, the patient and his or her family should still have the right to fund life-extending care. After studying the Constitution and the nation's legal foundations, I have concluded *all* these ideas, including the one I proposed, are patently offensive to the human condition. Simply put, neither government nor entity can be allowed to determine the circumstances by which funding of healthcare may be curtailed. I'll explain.

The United States was built on a previously unacknowledged set of principles; namely that human life is infinitely superior to government. Of all God's creations, we are the only creatures graced with the likeness of God. This unique attribute separates us from all other living beings and imparts upon each of us a direct and immutable relationship with the Creator. Consequently, neither king, nor man, nor government may interfere with our relationship with God, nor are they in positions to assess the value of our existence. After all, how can king, man, or government assess that which is infinitely and inconceivably valuable?

For this reason, government exists to support the people, not the other way around. Government can thus never be placed in the position of deciding the value of an innocent human life, or the merit of discarding it. Viewed differently, if government is placed in a position to decide on withdrawing a person's care, then by definition, it is being done under the presumption that human life is somehow subservient to the government's judgment, a position irreconcilably incompatible with the precepts of America's foundation.

In fact, we have already witnessed the revolting consequences of the abandonment of man's divinity as a check on power. In 2013, eleven-year-old Sarah Murnaghan was dying from cystic fibrosis. As is the natural course of the disease, her lungs were relentlessly failing, causing her to barely have enough air to live. Doctors tried everything to spare the young girl's life. They were down to their last option: lung transplant. The problem was that people under the age of twelve, by policy of the Organ Procurement and Transplantation

Network (OPTN), were prohibited from receiving a lung transplant pursuant to the "Under 12 Rule."[286] The bases for the prohibition were largely centered on the size of an eleven-year-old's lungs compared to the size of an adult set of lungs and the lack of available data on the survivability of such young candidates. But Sarah's doctors thought she was physiologically capable of tolerating an adult set of lungs in transplantation.

As the battle raged within administrative circles, Sarah's life was slowly slipping away from her. By May 2013, Sarah had about 5 weeks to live.[287] Amazingly, and most offensively, because Congress implemented the United Network for Organ Sharing, which runs the OPTN, the decision of whether Sarah would live or die ultimately fell upon SecHHS. In this case, SecHHS was Kathleen Sebelius, a liberal progressive.[xxiv]

Sebelius's position was that making an exception for Sarah allowing her to participate in the adult lung transplant program would potentially hurt another who could receive the transplant. By her decision, Sebelius essentially was sentencing little Sarah to death. The case would ultimately make its way to the judiciary, which stayed Sebelius's decision and allowed Sarah to receive her lung transplant.[288]

Despite a series of early complications, Sarah ultimately thrived. In 2018, Sarah was a ninth-grade honors student who helped her mother write a book entitled *Saving Sarah: One Mother's Battle against the Healthcare System to Save Her Daughter's Life* and traveled with her to promote the book.[289]

[xxiv] This is the same Kathleen Sebelius who thought it within her authority to teach Americans how they should cover their mouths while sneezing. Victor, Daniel, "Sneeze into Your Elbow, Not Your Hand. Please," *The New York Times* (blog), Feb. 27, 2018, accessed Aug. 2, 2019, https://www.nytimes.com/2018/02/27/health/how-to-sneeze.html.

Sarah's case inspired countless discussions regarding the ethics of allocating limited, life-saving, medical resources. Relatively absent amongst these discussions is the appropriateness of placing a government that is subservient to the people in a position of ending the life of a human being who has not been convicted of perpetrating a heinous crime.[xxv]

Another disturbing case is that of Terri Schiavo in Florida. Terri was a married young woman who suffered a heart attack in her home on February 25, 1990, when she was only 26 years old. She was found pulseless, but through heroic life-saving efforts, paramedics were able to resuscitate her and transport her to the hospital alive. Terri, who had suffered from bulimia, had lost over 100 pounds prior to marrying Michael Schiavo. Her collapse was likely the result of a poor diet, which appeared to cause her to become dangerously hypokalemic.[xxvi, 290]

Initially in a coma, Terri eventually entered into a permanent, severely brain-damaged state such that she relied on others for the most essential biological functions including drinking and feeding. She persisted in that vegetative state for years. On June 18, 1990, her husband was appointed her legal guardian.[291] Michael tried every reasonable option to restore his wife to a more interactive state including taking Terri to California to implant an experimental thalamic stimulator.[292] Mr. Schiavo even successfully prosecuted a

---

[xxv] The death penalty is a situation where government ultimately makes the decision over the end of someone's life and carries out its extermination. The discussion regarding the death penalty is obviously outside the scope of healthcare policy and thus is not entertained here. Suffice it to say here, that one convicted of a heinous crime is not an innocent player, but a criminal with a debt to society and to his or her victims. Mine is not to defend the death penalty in this footnote, but merely to point out the difference between government's role in withholding care from a sick or injured individual and executing a convicted heinous criminal.

[xxvi] Hypokalemia is a condition where one has an excessively low potassium level. An essential mineral, no one can survive without potassium.

medical malpractice lawsuit against Terri's doctors that resulted in the creation of a trust fund of about $1 million.[293]

Throughout this time, Michael worked closely with Terri's mother, Mary Schindler in caring for Terri and in arranging for her medical treatments. But in 1994, that relationship changed when Michael decided the best course was to discontinue treatment and allow Terri to pass.[294] Michael averred that his wife would not wish to live in a permanently dependent state and began the long judicial process to have her feeding tube removed.

Terri's parents were adamantly opposed to the idea of letting Terri go and actively fought Michael in his efforts to discontinue medical, nutritional, and hydrational support for Terri. In 1998, an independent evaluator opined that the views expressed by Terri when she had capacity were "not clear and convincing, . . . [and that] . . . potential conflicts of interest regarding the disposition of the residual funds in Theresa's trust account" existed.[xxvii, 295]

In 2001, Terri's feeding tube was removed, but was later reconnected. Subsequently, court battle after court battle was decided in favor of Michael's efforts at removing Terri's feeding tube, and by extension, of hastening her death. Moved by the direction the judiciary was steering this case, the Florida legislature, convened in special session on October 21, 2003, and authorized Governor Jeb Bush to stay the judicial order to disconnect Terri's feeding tube, which the governor obeyed that the same day.[296] Michael Schiavo challenged "Terri's Law" before the Florida Supreme Court with the assistance of the ACLU, and the Court ruled the law to be unconstitutional.

[xxvii] Significantly, by 2005, the time when Terri's tube was finally and permanently pulled, Michael was living with another woman with whom he had already fathered two children. Wesley J. Smith, "The Left's Continuing Lies about the Terri Schiavo Case," *National Review* (blog), June 11, 2019, accessed on Aug. 12, 2019, https://www.nationalreview.com/corner/lefts-continuing-lies-about-the-terri-schiavo-case/.

On March 18, 2005, Terri's feeding tube was removed in com-pliance with a court order. This time it was Congress that entered into a special session and passed the "Palm Sunday Compromise" authorizing federal courts to review the case *de novo*.[xxviii] President Bush signed the legislation at 1:11 am on March 21, 2005, allowing the federal court to review the case. Terri's parents' motions were ultimately denied, and the Supreme Court refused to hear the case, sealing Terri's fate.

Terri Schiavo lived 13 days without her feeding tube before she succumbed to dehydration on March 31, 2005. After her death, President Bush lamented, "The essence of civilization is that the strong have a duty to protect the weak. In cases where there are serious doubts and questions, the presumption should be in favor of life."[297] The Terri Schiavo case served as a defining moment in American society, and once again, lost in the conversation, was the evaluation of the ominous power of government and whether it, and in particular the federal government, should be given the authority to seal the death of an innocent.[xxix]

More examples of the government's ability to seal the fate of the innocent through healthcare decisions can be encountered in for-eign cases. One such case involved Charlie Gard, an eight-month-old child living in England. Baby Charlie suffered from a rare genetic disorder affecting his mitochondria.[xxx] By most accounts, Baby Charlie's condition was imminently fatal. Treating physicians

---

[xxviii] *De novo*: Under a new look. Without the influence of other court rulings.

[xxix] Once again, the term "innocent" is used here to highlight the fact that the deci-sion in Terri's case was not made in response to her committing a heinous act. Her death sentence served as neither retribution nor punishment for having murdered another or her having committed an atrocious act against humanity. She was sentenced to death merely because she had a chronic condition and no capacity to decide for herself what her fate should be.

[xxx] Mitochondria DNA depletion syndrome.

concluded that nothing else could be done to prolong the child's life, and even if there were, it would not provide Charlie with any chance at what they deemed to be a reasonable existence. The British physicians, against the family's wishes, decided that the most appropriate course was to withdraw care.

But Charlie's parents wished to continue to fight for their child's life, and they turned their attention to the United States where at least two doctors working on experimental treatments relating to Charlie's condition estimated a 10% chance their treatment could help.[298] Like the Schiavo and Murnaghan cases before it, Baby Charlie's struggles captured the hearts of millions around the world with over £1.2 million raised to transport him to the United States and fund his experimental care in the United States. Despite this gracious act of public benevolence essentially absolving the British government of any financial burden, it blocked the parents from exercising their inherent right to take Baby Charlie to a country that was willing and able to provide novel and experimental treatment because, according to British authorities, such treatment was not in the best interest of the child.[299]

According to one unidentified physician treating Baby Charlie, the British healthcare system was superior to that of the United States because if an intervention was not "in the child's best interest," the treatment would not be administered in England. But, the physician argued, "in America, provided parents have the money, the financial means to access care, doctors will do anything parents would like to be done regardless of what is happening to the child."[300]

Although the comment was aimed at demeaning American healthcare, it exemplified the greatness of American culture with one correction. There is no good-standing, American physician who would "do anything parents would like to be done regardless of what is happening to the child." Recall that American physicians take an oath to always do what's best for their patients. American physicians provide care only when indicated and then only when the potential benefits of the care provided outweigh its risks. But the unnamed British physician is correct in stating that American physicians would administer the care to the child even if governmental medical authorities "don't consider something to be in the child's best interest." And rightly so! In the United States, parents retain the ultimate authority regarding the appropriateness of proposed treatments for their children

One of the precepts of the United States implicitly ingrained in the Constitution is the supremacy of parenting rights over governmental desires. Unless a practice or intervention causes harm to a child or is abusive or threatening to the child's health or wellbeing the government is not permitted to interfere with the parents' decision. This is a far different standard from one holding that actions may only be taken if the *government* determines that the action, or treatment, is in the best interest of the child. In the former, it is the parent who prevails, unless harm is being done to the child. In the latter, as in England, it is the government that prevails, period. In the United States, as a matter of human rights, it is *precisely the parents* who get to decide what is in the child's best interest, not the government. To allow otherwise is to abdicate an essential precept of human autonomy and dignity, something Americans thus far have not been inclined to do.

Indeed, the difference between the care in the United States and that in England is that in England, even if the family raised the funds to help their son, government could stop them from fighting for their child's life. In the United States, government is still required to have sufficient respect for individual rights so that it could not. Once again, one cannot claim that a government is of the people, by the people, or for the people, if it gets to decide whether a child lives or dies despite the interests of the child's parents.

Baby Charlie died in England on July 28, 2017.[301]

Healthcare Rationing

If deciding whether a particular person gets to live or die is offensive, then it must naturally shock the conscience if those decisions were made regarding many. Such is the case where government interferes with a population's access to certain types of care, a process called rationing. Rationing is perhaps the most complicated aspect of healthcare policy because it is so ambiguous in scope that practically any decision, whether it is made by the patient or by anyone else, can be considered a form of rationing.

"Rationing" is "the act of distributing by allotting or apportioning [of healthcare] according to a plan."[302] In rationing, those allocating or apportioning resources are external to the individual affected. The government decides you cannot access something, or a committee decides it will not expend resources upon its constituency despite the desires of certain individuals. Although some have called the exercise of personal discretion in pursuing treatments "rationing," such personal decisions cannot qualify as rationing because they result in act of individualized discretion undertaken *by the individual* based on value considerations relative to resources available *to the individual*. Such personal decisions are fundamental to free market valuations. Further, since no person or entity is imposing impediments upon the individual keeping him from being able to access care, such personal considerations do not fit the definition of rationing. To hold otherwise is to eviscerate the role of any decision refraining from purchasing a good or service.

Personal discretion, even if inhibited by financial constraints, is by far the most appropriate, ethical, and deferential method of making healthcare utilization decisions, as it is the only one that respects the dignity and independence of the individual while honoring his or her rights as a human being.

There are numerous forms through which rationing is employed, some more obvious than others.

The lowest level where rationing can take place is with the physician. Indeed, many policy designers have tried to make the physician the bulwark for rationing. This is wholly inappropriate. The physician is the sage overseer and adviser of the types of goods and services to be consumed by the patient. The relationship of the physician to the patient is that of his or her fiduciary, its faithful servant. It is up to the physician, using all her education, knowledge, and experience, to select the most appropriate healthcare products or services for her patient, ideally without regard for price or ability to pay. In fashioning a patient's treatment, the physician is not to consider population dynamics, resource allocations, or purposes other than the best interests of the patient. With her patient lies her only allegiance. It is therefore indefensible to place upon the physician any burden other than what is best for the patient. In fact, it is essential to the integrity of the patient-physician relationship that the doctor's allegiance rest squarely and entirely upon her patient as it is the only way the patient will know the advice being offered is best for him or her. Placing upon the physician considerations regarding what is best for the population or for society at the expense of the patient detracts, in fact, nullifies the very essence of the patient-physician relationship, the most valuable pillar in a healthcare delivery system.

Of course, the patient may bring up considerations of price, affordability, and reasonability, among others, to the physician. Under such circumstances, the physician is duty-bound to consider them with the patient and advise him or her accordingly. But when the patient entertains such factors, it is the patient, rightfully, who is the final arbiter of the feasibility, affordability, and value of the purchase, not anyone else.

The third-party payer, or the insurance company will ration. So long as the third-party payer is a private company, then, in theory at least, it is not the government that is rationing the care. But, whether it is the government or a private entity making the decisions that impede access, the patient's ability to make the final value judgment on whether to pursue the care being offered is thwarted.

There are many methods by which insurance companies ration care, most of them mirroring governmental techniques. An insurer may refuse to cover a service, making it unfeasible for the patient to access it on her own. It may delay its delivery. It may place the proposed service under the scrutiny of an arbiter under the insurer's payroll or authority who decides whether the service is worth it or not, *to the insurer*! Or it may limit access to the care being sought. In either case, the insurer's priority is not the value of the treatment to the patient, but to the insurer's bottom line.

Healthcare insurance is a business, and like any other business venture, its goal is to generate money for itself and its investors. The decisions made by the private insurer are not guided by the patient's health, altruistic as any one insurer's vision may be. Ultimately, the third-party payer's decisions must strike a balance between avoiding litigation, gaining a firm hold on the marketplace, and generating capital. And in its hierarchy, the latter controls the former two. Under this scheme, the patient plays a very small role in the policy-making priorities for the insurer, causing the patient to feel powerless over the decisions regarding his or her care.

Ultimately, there is but one power play the patient has when disagreeing with an insurance company's policy decision: to seek another insurer. This power play disappears when it is government that controls the strings. If the government rations, there is no escaping the policy because it applies to everyone. There is no second opinion because there is no competitor from which to get it. And even in a democratic society, there may be no appealing the policy because it is formulated in a bureaucratic desk by some non-elected official hidden deep within the bowels of some building in Maryland. This latter scenario may seem far-fetched, but it is actually what routinely transpires today in the Medicare program, and is exactly what the Left hoped to accomplish through IPAB.[xxxi]

Recall that in creating IPAB under the Obama Administration, Congress crafted a panel, immune from questioning by Congress, the judiciary, or the individual patient, regarding reimbursements made to providers for certain medical interventions. The structure was so offensive that despite Congress's inefficiencies and dysfunctions, it was able to reverse itself on this policy and permanently eradicate the Board...for now. Nevertheless, its creation heralded two priorities for those seeking the implementation of a centralized healthcare delivery system. First, it spoke of the Left's wanton desire to make decisions regarding the survivability of individuals without regard for their opinions or priorities, and second, it fully displayed the audacity with which these proponents were willing to control the lives of others.

[xxxi] See pages 68-71

But as hinted in addressing rationing techniques employed by third-party payers, government possesses a plethora of methods through which it may ration the care delivered to its constituents. The most obvious of these is the prohibition.

Rationing by direct prohibition is very difficult to accomplish in the United States. Here, reference is not made to the prohibition of accessing a product because it is too dangerous or because there is no identified beneficial medical application. What I am referring to is the prohibition against accessing a product or medication known to have a beneficial role in the treatment or prevention of disease simply because it is too expensive or difficult to supply to the public.

In the United States, thanks to the constitutional restrictions placed upon government, once a product is deemed beneficial, it is nearly impossible to explicitly prohibit its use. Instead, government employs other methods of limiting its access. The most prevalent of these is price controls. If government can control the reimbursement of certain items or services, it places itself in the position of being able to determine the items and services to which the public has access. This was a primary motivator behind IPAB, and as we shall see, it was a weapon made possible through Medicare's prohibition on balance billing.

Delaying access to care is another very effective method for rationing, and here, Canada likely serves as the best example. As of 2017, over one million Canadians found themselves waiting for necessary treatments, the first time the greater than 1 million figure had been reached.[303] What's more, the median wait for treatment by a specialist in Canada is 21 weeks, the longest ever recorded for that country.[304] Of course, the protracted waits are not without deleterious consequences as between 1,591 and 3,943 people die each year in Canada due to the delay in care. And these estimates are based on numbers spanning 1993 through 2009 when the volume of patients waiting and the magnitude of their delays were shorter than they are presently![305]

The situation in England is no better where the methods employed are even more authoritarian. England has the largest single-payer system in the world, the National Health Service (NHS)[306] and is frustrated by the inescapable quagmire inherent to centralized healthcare: political agendas. The NHS Constitution states that it "provides a comprehensive service available to all,"[307] but it also cautions that it "has a wider social duty to promote equality through the services it provides and to pay particular attention to groups or sections of society where improvements in health and life expectancy are not keeping pace with the rest of the population."[308] The offensiveness of this latter sentence is overwhelming as the British government is openly expressly that it treats certain people differently from others. And although the same constitution states that "[t]he patient will be at the heart of everything it does,"[309] it also states, "The NHS is committed to providing the best value for *taxpayers'* money."[310] (Emphasis added.) So, what exactly is at the heart of the NHS's concern, the patient, or the taxpayer? The NHS Constitution provides us with the answer to that question as well in stating, "We accept that difficult decisions have to be taken-that when we waste resource we waste opportunities for others."[311]

Clearly, the answer is the NHS's priorities lie with the wellbeing of "others," not necessarily with that of the individual patient.

The result of placing such dual allegiances in healthcare prioritization is that patients often do not get the services they need due to decisions made by the government, i.e. rationing. For example, in 2019, the NHS decided to reduce funding for cataract surgery causing many patients to wait months for surgeries available within weeks or days in the United States.[312] Others faced artificially contrived eligibility restrictions prohibiting them from accessing the procedure even though the surgery was medically indicated.

Indeed, the manner through which England arrives at its rationing decisions is Orwellian, to say the least. In 1999, the National Institute for Health and Clinical Experience (NICE) was created to manage healthcare expenditure allocations. But its acronym defies the organization's dehumanizing policies. Essentially, NICE has decided that human life is only worth salvaging if the treatment provided results in more than £50,000 of value per quality-adjusted year.[313] This is even harsher than may appear at first blush because, under this policy, the yearly expenditure must be corrected by the value of the life achieved! For example, if a cancer treatment costs £30,000 per year, but the person's life during that time is so painful that its value, as estimated by the government, is only 50% of perfect health, the expenditure is corrected by half, making the quality-adjusted, yearly expenditure of the treatment £60,000 per quality-adjusted year.[xxxii] The life-saving/extending treatment is, therefore, more expensive than the arbitrarily contrived £50,000 per quality-adjusted year, and NICE will deny the treatment.[314]

That England, one of the world's leading democracies, should implement such a harsh and inhumane system should be a chilling warning to any constituency considering giving its government similarly broad authorities regarding healthcare.

This brings us the biggest fallacy of all: single-payer healthcare is free! This is an outright lie promoted not only by advocates of

---

[xxxii] £30,000 per year/0.5 quality adjustment years=£60,000 per quality-adjusted years.

universal healthcare, but also by the governments purporting to provide it.

The British NHS Constitution reads, "NHS services are free of charge, except in limited circumstances sanctioned by Parliament."[315] The truth is that NHS's services are not free of charge. Like all other commodities, they have a price. In England, in fiscal year 2018-2019, the expenditures for the Department of Health and Social Care in England were £132.9 billion,[316] or £2,389.43 per English person.[xxxiii] That figure assumes equal payments by everyone, rich or poor, able to pay, or not.[xxxiv]

In the United States, government rationing of healthcare takes on a much more sophisticated approach than pure fiat or the direct restriction of the availability of services. To put it simply, the federal government uses price incentives in support of market trends it favors and to obstruct those it does not. We have seen this time and again on a myriad of issues. For example, in regulating Medicare, Congress relies on the Medicare Payment Advisory Board (Med-PAC). This governmental agency is chartered with the responsibility of "analyzing access to care, quality of care, and other issues affecting Medicare."[317] In other words, rationing.

True, the directive does not expressly employ the word "rationing," but advising Congress regarding "access to care" with the express purpose of establishing policies affecting that access is the very

---

[xxxiii] Based on a population of 55.62 million people in England.

[xxxiv] Government financed health expenditures account for 79% of all healthcare spending in England. Consequently, total healthcare expenditures in England are estimated at £2,989 per capita. "Healthcare Expenditure, UK Health Accounts 2017," Office for National Statistics, accessed on Sept. 7, 2019, https://www.ons.gov.uk/peoplepopulationandcommunity/healthandsocialcare/healthcaresystem/bulletins/ukhealthaccounts/2017. In the United States, the per capita healthcare expenditure is $10,739 per person. "Historical," CMS.gov, accessed on Sept. 6, 2019, https://www.cms.gov/Research-Statistics-Data-and-Systems/Statistics-Trends-and-Reports/NationalHealthExpendData/NationalHealthAccountsHistorical.html.

definition of rationing. MedPAC is made up of 17 members "with national recognition for their expertise in health finance and economics, actuarial science, health facility management, health plans, and integrated delivery systems, reimbursement of health facilities, allopathic and osteopathic physicians, and other providers of health services, and other related fields, who provide a mix of different professionals, broad geographic representation, and a balance between urban and rural representatives."[318] These members are appointed by the Comptroller General whose selections are limited only by the requirement that the selected Commissioners have expertise in healthcare and that the majority be non-healthcare providers.[319]

Predictably, MedPAC routinely engages in discussions regarding the methods by which the federal government should inject itself into the healthcare market to interfere with the administration of that care to better fit the Commissioners' vision. Not only do these considerations overtly cross the threshold into the arena of rationing, but also they widely exceed the authorities conferred to the federal government under Article I of the Constitution of the United States. In effect, MedPAC attempts to conceal its healthcare rationing function by claiming they are preventing "overutilization," or ensuring "payment accuracy," "cost efficiency," "quality of care," and "resource allocation."

Take for instance MedPac's manipulation of emergency room services. In its April 4, 2018, meeting, MedPAC voted to advise Congress to cut reimbursements to freestanding emergency rooms operating within 6 miles of their parent hospitals by 30%.[320] Its reason, as expressed in its subsequent report to Congress, was that "the policy would reduce the incentive to develop new [stand-alone emergency departments] in close proximity to on-campus hospital EDs."[321] Here, MedPAC brazenly and openly admitted injecting itself into the decision-making rubric for hospitals considering opening freestanding emergency rooms and acknowledged that their "payment system for emergency room services would encourage providers to treat lower intensity patients in emergency rooms rather than at urgent care centers."[322]

But what business is it of MedPAC or any other federal agency to be advising the hospital, much less pressuring it into making market feasibility decisions? MedPAC argued that because stand-alone emergency rooms tend to treat lower intensity patients they should be paid at a lower level, and that six miles seemed to be an appropriate distance in which to enforce these reimbursement cuts.[323] Not lost to MedPAC was the fact that the reimbursement cuts would save Medicare over $250 million annually.[324]

Hospitals may have countless other valid reasons to build a freestanding emergency room near their primary facility. What if the hospital wanted to alleviate the waiting times in their primary emergency room by building a second facility nearby? What if the hospital was concerned over the travel distance to the primary facility from its stand-alone facility and aimed to limit that risk through proximity? Or what if the hospital simply saw a money-making opportunity based on the local market demands it was identifying? Bear in mind that many of the facilities MedPAC is regulating have already been built, and the decisions to invest in their construction have already been made. With its decision, MedPAC changed the assumptions regarding facility investment and construction efforts. MedPAC's decision to disturb the operations of stand-alone emergency rooms affected 25%[325] of the country's 550-600 stand-alone emergency rooms,[326] translating to the suppression by fiat of innumerable opportunities to alleviate long waiting room times, of potential decrease travel distances for patients, and of a slew of partially finished construction projects that will never be completed.

But stand-alone emergency rooms are not the only forum where MedPAC and the federal government have pulled their stunts. In 2007, CHS implemented a series of incremental reimbursement cuts for procedures performed in freestanding cardiology suites. In all, reimbursements to those freestanding facilities were cut by 47%, a level less than the cost of performing them.[327] With only about 100 such centers operating in the United States in 2007,[328] these cuts resulted in the closure of outpatient cardiac catheterization facilities and a precipitous decrease in the number of cardiac catheterizations performed in outpatient centers.[329] Concurrently, CMS inexplicably allotted a 25% increase in reimbursements for the same procedures performed in hospital settings.[330]

So, why would MedPAC change these reimbursement formulas to favor hospitals over freestanding facilities? Being that there is no objective policy advantage for such a move, the one logical answer for its introduction is the Commission's bias. Take, for example, MedPAC's position on physician-owned specialty hospitals. These facilities are primarily owned by physicians and provided inpatient care in only certain specific areas of medicine. One facility may only provide cardiothoracic care. Another may limit itself to orthopaedics, and yet another to cancer patients. Physician-owned specialty hospitals tend to be associated with improved outcomes, higher quality of care, and shorter inpatient stays. In fact, in 2005, MedPAC released a report to Congress on physician-owned specialty hospitals where it confirmed their favorable outcomes and the absence of any negative effects upon their communities by their presence.[331]

Despite these findings, MedPAC recommended reimbursements for general, acute care hospital be increased at the expense of specialty hospitals for identical procedures. Amazingly, its rationale was that physician-owned specialty hospitals were too profitable![332] In a follow-up report, MedPAC also objected to a doubling in the number of physician-owned specialty hospitals between 2002 and 2004 and a 6% increase in cardiac surgery performed in communities with physician-owned cardiac hospitals.[333] In one of its most hostile comments, MedPAC stated that these facilities were "diverting patients from competitor community hospitals"[334] as if those patients belonged to those facilities in the first place. Ironically, since that time, the organic push in the medical industry has been to simplify procedures and make them less invasive such that now it is technology, progress, and innovation that is "diverting patients" away from hospitals with predicted savings of over $2 billion per year.[335] With its market interferences, MedPAC only served to impede what patients and technology were going to eventually require, and diminished the economic efficiency with which the transition was made.

MedPAC's decisions also impact the diagnoses made on patients and their rendered treatments. Osteoporosis, or the thinning of one's bones, is known as a silent killer because it is a painless, imperceptible process that leads to fractures. The condition mostly afflicts older patients and in particular, postmenopausal women.

Dual x-ray absorptiometry (DXA) is the principal way of identifying osteoporotic patients. In the United States alone, approximately 53.6 million adults suffer from osteoporosis, whether they are aware of the condition or not.[336] People with osteoporosis are approximately 7 times more likely to develop hip fractures than their similarly aged cohorts.[337] Identifying patients with osteoporosis using screening tests like the DXA scan is therefore paramount to fracture prevention.

Initially, a large number of DXA scans were done in physicians' offices. In fact, in 2002, 70% of all DXA scans were performed in the office setting.[338] But beginning in 2007, MedPAC and CMS implemented a series of cuts on office-performed DXA reimbursements such that payments received for DXA scans performed in a non-facility setting (a physician's office) were 63% lower by 2010. Medical offices stopped performing the procedures because the costs of performing these procedures were greater than the reimbursement offered by Medicare.[339] As a result, in 2008, 3,680,948 fewer DXA scans were performed that year, and 43,661 more hip fractures occurred at a cost of $1.8 billion to Medicare[340] and an increase of 9,418 fracture-related deaths.[341]

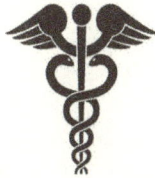

Chapter 6

Free Market Solutions to America's Healthcare Challenges

The most powerful engine propelling innovation, availability, and access is the free market. That a person is free to dream of a better life, conjure an idea to improve human existence, and profit from it while elevating himself or herself to a higher level of comfort and socioeconomic status is a steeple of American society and culture. It stems from America's deep respect for property rights and reward through personal achievement. These forces that have worked so well for society in general, function equally as well for healthcare. Therefore, they ought to be harnessed, both for society's benefit and for the wellbeing of individuals. But before considering how to do this, it is important to define exactly what is meant by a free market system as it applies to healthcare.

As opposed to a socialist healthcare system where government owns and controls the means of production and distribution of healthcare-related goods and services, a free market healthcare delivery system is one where the various goods and services are privately owned, and their exchanges are undertaken freely, subject to prices independently agreed upon by patients and providers without intervention from outside parties, especially government. In a free market healthcare system, the terms of the exchange arrived at by the seller and the consumer are driven by the relative supply and demand of that product or service. The free market is the ideal system of interaction and price-setting because the actual participants are in full control of the delivery of the care they seek. They alone are responsible for the development of a treatment plan. And most importantly, they alone determine the value of the product being offered.

Admittedly, there are factors inherent to healthcare preventing a pure, free market healthcare system from functioning. First, some exchanges between the consumer and the provider are not discretionary. When someone suddenly develops chest pain and shortness of breath along with feelings of impending doom or death, he is not in a position to engage in a negotiation over the terms governing the delivery of his care. The gravity of the situation and the dire consequences of not agreeing to the necessary treatment make his position in negotiating untenable. Under these circumstances, the consumer would be willing to pay *anything* for his treatment. Simply put, the patient and provider are not on equal footing making it impossible for them to freely negotiate the terms of the exchange. Even if an alleged agreement were reached, it would carry no moral or legal weight since the seller (the healthcare provider) held all the advantages over the consumer, and the buyer (the patient) had no leverage with which to negotiate. He either accepts the terms imposed upon him or risks dying. In short, there was no opportunity to foster a meeting of the minds relating to the terms of the exchange.

Similar considerations prevail, of course, for the patient who lacks capacity and needs urgent or emergent treatment. Suppose our unfortunate heart attack patient is also unconscious. How could he possibly engage in contract negotiations? Is he then left to die? Under a pure free market system, the absurd result would be that he would.

Another challenge is the tension between those who cannot pay and America's moral commitment to the wellbeing of all. In all societies, capitalist or otherwise, there exists poverty. As such, poor individuals will be in no position to purchase the healthcare services they need to allow them to continue functioning. In a purely free market system, those who are destitute would be unable to pay for any healthcare services. I was confronted with this situation during my service in the early 1990s when I was assigned, as a flight surgeon, to a makeshift encampment in Somalia. We were placed in a tent in the devastated streets of Mogadishu and tasked with treating anyone who may seek care. On one occasion, a Somali woman was brought to me in a wheel barrel for treatment. She was suffering from pneumonia and was so weakened by her affliction that her head painfully bounced off the back edge of the wheel barrel as it made its way through countless bumps on the unpaved ground. She was febrile, terribly dehydrated and her lungs full of infectious secretions that would gurgle as she breathed.

With her husband's aid, we brought her to our tent, laid her on a cot, and began rehydrating her while we treated her with intravenous antibiotics. This unfortunate woman was at death's door when she arrived, but with the most rudimentary of care, forty-eight hours later, she was able to walk to her home with her husband and a pocketful of oral antibiotics with which to complete her treatment.

I recall asking her husband what he would have done had we, the American military, not been there. He told me his wife would have died because there was nowhere else to go.

But couldn't he have taken her to the hospital? I asked.

He laughed as he answered me through an interpreter. "If you have no money, they will not help you," he said. "If I had brought her in my wheel barrel to the front door of the hospital without money, they would not have let her in. They would have let her die right there, at their front steps."

It is difficult to pass judgment on a destitute nation like Somalia, but certainly, no American would accept a system where a fellow citizen would die at a hospital's front door merely because he is unable to pay for his care. This is where the nation's Christian makeup and the charitable character of its people come into play. The American people, in their benevolence and inherent goodwill, will always demand a stopgap to the slippery slide into misery and death of its most vulnerable.

Another shortcoming of a pure free market healthcare system is the absence of any accommodation for public health. This is because the motivations for purchases under a pure free market system are driven by the needs of the individual, not by the collective needs of a population. Activities designed for the betterment of the health of the population require individual members of that population to expend energy or resources, not for their individual improvement, but for that of everyone else. It is true that each individual will ultimately benefit from these activities, but the gains are not directly linked to the individual and are ones that require a relatively large investment to prevent an uncertain occurrence.

The state could adopt a myriad of public health policy interventions. It may require all to receive certain vaccinations. It may limit the practice of medicine to certain individuals who maintain certain qualifications. It may prohibit the use of certain medications, or require compliance with certain measures to run a hospital. We saw these types of government interventions implemented as far back as America's colonial period via quarantine legislation, mandatory smallpox vaccinations, and the imposition of licensure requirements for the practice of medicine. But merely because the government undertakes interventions to regulate some aspects of healthcare and to promote the public's health does not in and of itself make its healthcare system something other than a free market based system.

To uphold such a free market system there are several provisions with which government must comply. First, it cannot select a particular vendor or favor a specific market participant over another. Second, it cannot manipulate prices. Third, those interventions government finds necessary to implement must be as minimally invasive as possible. And finally, they must be legislated at a level closest to the constituents. A free market healthcare system simply must ensure that the exchange of goods and services, with rare exceptions, be undertaken independently by patients and providers with minimal intervention from outside parties. It must also guarantee that individuals remain free to independently pursue, to the greatest extent possible, their respective opportunities for treatment.

There *are* free market solutions to the healthcare problems confronting us today, and they do not rely on the centralization of America's healthcare system or on the acquisition of our decision-making authority by government. Quite the opposite. The solutions for our healthcare are ones that keep the decisions regarding our health under our control as individuals. They are ideas and enactments observing the dignity of each individual, allowing for innovation, and tapping into our basic human desire for self-improvement and self-preservation.

One other point is important here, namely the realization that the United States does not possess a unified healthcare policy.

Instead, our "healthcare delivery system" consists of an assortment of silos, each working independently of the other. There is a Medicare system run by the federal government to provide coverage to our nation's senior citizens. There is a veterans' system covering our nation's military veterans. There is the military healthcare system designed to care for our nation's active-duty personnel and their families. The Indian Health Service provides personal and public health services to the nation's American Indian and Alaskan Native populations. Medicaid aids the poor and the disabled through the actions of the various states while being largely funded and controlled by the federal government. The ERISA system is regulated by the federal government and has jurisdiction over insurance products provided by large employers. And then there is the collapsing Obamacare system, which served only to coerce the nation's insurers into funding the care Washington deemed necessary and to force citizens into buying insurance whether they wanted to or not. The remainder of healthcare, including private insurance products, is regulated by the various states, each with its nuances and peculiarities.

With this cacophony of regulatory silos working in relative isolation, there is no credible argument to be made regarding the existence of a coordinated healthcare system in America. There is no overall plan governing how these various systems interact and complement each other. Medicare rules do not apply to Medicaid. The Indian Health Service operates markedly differently from the VA system. Physicians and health providers recognized as competent in one system are not recognized as such in another. And there is no interchangeability between the insurance products active in one state and those active in another. These regionalisms and legal hurdles only serve to stymie competition, establish regional oligopolies, suppress innovation, and promote higher premiums and costs.

What we need is to establish a legal and economic framework within which our nation's greatest minds, those people driven to serve others through the delivery of healthcare products and services, are motivated to dream, follow through on their vision, and if useful to the public, capitalize on their ideas. Instead, what we have been doing is to task the government with the creation of a vast array of discombobulated, nearly incomprehensible laws and regulations serving only to depress the human spirit and to remove the decision-making authority from the very people this uniquely American system of government is supposed to serve.

We have seen many examples of just how government intervention serves to diminish the greatness and responsiveness of the nation's healthcare delivery. We have encountered this in the United States with the difficulties in accessing care posed by the VA, IHS, and Medicaid systems. And before heaping praise upon Medicare as a shining exception to the overall rule, recall that Medicare, through its price regulations and its influences in consolidating local and regional healthcare systems has served to manipulate the delivery of services in a manner commensurate with its interests, not necessarily the interests of its beneficiaries. And Medicare has its own sustainability issues since it is expected to go bankrupt by 2026.[342]

The reality is that only one person or entity can look out for your best interests when making considerations regarding your treatment. That entity is you. Whenever government or any other party takes control of your healthcare, the decisions made stop being those necessarily in your best interest. Instead, issues such as budgeting constraints, return on investment projections, resource management considerations, and future expense fears lead to the implementation of provisions contrary to your best interests. And when you feel it necessary to fight back, there are precious few places for you to go to decisions made about your health reconsidered. Instead, the road to the care you need becomes a dead-end street.

So where does the answer to the future of our nation's healthcare system lie? Quite simply, it lies with you and in transferring as much autonomy regarding your health and your healthcare to you as possible. Instead of centralizing the system and placing decisions at the hands of bureaucrats and politicians, we should be aiming to place healthcare decisions and its consequences in your hands. Doing so would minimize the risk of our healthcare being withheld from you. It will minimize the opportunities of being rationed out of accessing care, and it will, with more predictability than any other system, provide a favorable environment for reducing your healthcare costs, as well as our collective expenditures.

What follows is a description of how such a system would look.

Healthcare Is Not a Right

The first consideration is the acknowledgment that healthcare is not a right. It is a commodity, like any other. A right is something to which one has a just claim.[343] Healthcare does not remotely fit this definition. Specifically, no one can exert a "just claim" on healthcare. Healthcare is distinctively not like ownerless land to which one may lay a claim by working it or possessing it. Healthcare is also not like one's thoughts or beliefs that can be created, organized, and delivered merely through one's efforts and contemplations. Instead, healthcare exists and is delivered through the efforts of others. Merely because one is sick does not give one the authority to demand that a doctor, nurse, or any other healthcare practitioner slave over another to ensure one's prompt and complete recovery. Nor do those providers magically appear at one's bedside to provide the demanded care. For these individuals to even be in a position to help they have to go through years of labor and toil developing the prerequisite skills, knowledge, and expertise in their respective fields. The cost to them in energy and time is irreplaceable, and it is no one's right to take their skills from them by fiat.

Nor are these individuals required to gratuitously provide their services to the injured or infirmed merely because they have acquired the requisite skills to do so. If there is anyone who has a claim to anything in this scenario, it is the provider who has the right to possess, deliver, or withhold his or her skills, knowledge, and experience as she sees fit. The provider owns those skills because she has developed them through the power of her labor. She is the rightful owner and possessor of those skills. If the medical student wishes to go through the trouble of graduating from medical school merely to not practice medicine a single day of his or her life, that is his or her prerogative; not yours, not governments, or anyone else's. In a free and just society, one cannot demand that a professional deliver to another his or her services as a matter of right. This concept is nonsensical, oppressive, and unjust. However disdainful it may sound to the Left, healthcare is a product, which like happiness, one only has the right to pursue.

What makes healthcare different from most other commodities is its intimate ties to the moral obligation many of us feel to help others, particularly the infirmed. But these moral obligations do not confer upon anyone the right to demand that any other act in a certain way. By their very nature, these moral obligations are ones we place upon ourselves in service to God. However wonderful it may be that any of us devotes our lives to caring for the sick, whether for profit or sacrifice, it still does not create a right upon anyone to demand us to do so.

But even though healthcare is not anyone's to demand by right, or to distribute by fiat, its expanse is so intimate and so closely juxtaposed to human existence–namely the care and maintenance of our bodies–that a loyal and reverential respect for human dignity must remain as its centerpiece. This respect for human dignity does not equate to providing healthcare to every individual without impediments. Such a situation represents an impossibility because there will always be insufficient resources to provide all members of society with unlimited access to healthcare.

The requisite respect for human dignity necessitates that a just healthcare system honor, as much as is humanly possible, the decisions made by an individual regarding his healthcare and that he be provided with as much control as possible of the direction his care takes.

Some argue that because of the pressing nature of healthcare interactions and services, a level playing field does not exist between the negotiating parties. In reality, only about 10% of healthcare expenditures deal with emergency services.[344] It stands to reason then, that if 90% of the healthcare market is subject to measured free market influences, they should effectively and positively affect the healthcare industry, just as they do any other economic silo. The challenge before us, then, is not to devise methods by which products or services can be *demanded* from healthcare professionals, or how these market pressures may be bypassed. Rather it lies in the development of methods through which all may have the opportunity to pursue these resources and those interested in doing so may be motivated to delivering them.

Transforming the Way America Pays for Healthcare

For far too long, policymakers have focused on controlling the forces driving healthcare consumption rather than harnessing them. They have been preoccupied with controlling the nation's healthcare delivery instead of on allowing Americans to keep control of their care, particularly when they need it the most. Key in this effort is the enhancement of opportunities for patients to directly fund their care.

Presently, 53% of Americans are insured through private plans and another 36% through public sources.[345] Two insights can be obtained from these facts. First, so long as Americans remain dependent on third party payers for the funding of their healthcare, they will never achieve independence in determining the care they receive. Second, being that the percentage of Americans not funding for their care is so massive (at least 89%), a transition away from this third party dependence on healthcare funding will not take place overnight.

The key to establishing patient autonomy in funding healthcare is the health savings account (HSA). An HSA is a tax-deductible savings account managed by the patient and implemented to pay for the costs of healthcare. Through an HSA, the patient is in complete control of his or her care, from the treatment he or she accepts to the amount paid for it. No other system of healthcare payment offers a greater degree of autonomy and independence to the patient than the HSA.

Why aren't HSAs more frequently employed in paying for healthcare? The answer to that question, once again, is government interference. Presently, the tax code recognizes HSA eligibility only for those who are not enrolled in Medicare and possess a high deductible health plan (HDHP).[346] An HDHP is a healthcare insurance policy covering preventive services before the deductible and carrying a minimum deductible of $1,400 for an individual or $2,800 for a family.[347] Under such circumstances, the taxpayer is allowed to contribute up to $3,550 to his individual HSA, or up to $7,100 for family coverage.[348] When not used, the funds are allowed to roll over and earn interest, which is also not taxable.

The present model for HSA regulation is nowhere near ideal. Linking HSAs to specific insurance products only allows for the insurance company to benefit by favoring the sale of HDHPs and allowing them to become involved in a patient's decision-making process. Additionally, because HDHPs cover preventive medicine services before applying a deductible, the power of HSAs to curtail expenses is repressed. The advocate for this restrictive arrangement argues that HSAs discourage the taxpayer/beneficiary from spending money and therefore from seeking preventive medicine services, but *it is not the government's role to either encourage or coerce the people into seeking preventive healthcare services*. Additionally, the requirement of purchasing an HDHP before being eligible to fund an HSA robs valuable capital from the individual making decisions about her budget.

Another nonsensical and unproductive provision in the present HSA legislation is the exclusion of Medicare recipients from participating in HSAs. This restriction is particularly nonsensical as it targets the nation's principal healthcare consumers. Medicare enrollees have the greatest power to bend the spending curve and have the greatest resources available to spend on healthcare. They should be employed in the national effort to curb prices and make providers accountable to their patients.

And why would a person who is 65 years of age or older contribute to an HSA? Divisibility! The ability of the HSA's owner to will his funds to subsequent generations is the key factor in the long-term development of intergenerational financial independence in healthcare.

Indeed, the beneficial effects of HSAs to healthcare cost containment and efficiency is so great that shifting America's dependence away from health insurance and to HSAs should be a national priority. In fact, one estimate holds that shifting half of America's employer insurance policies to HSAs would result in cost savings of $57 billion per year![349] And another concluded that a complete transition to HSA based healthcare funding could save up to $400 billion per year.[350] After all we have seen and experienced with third-party directed healthcare, isn't it time we demanded this change from our policymakers?

The Elimination of Mandated Fee Schedules

We have seen how the implementation of a mandated fee schedule depresses market pressures and places an unacceptable amount of power at the hands of the third-party payer in determining the availability of products or services. These mandated fee schedules should be eliminated for nonurgent or nonemergent procedures or services. Instead, the third-party payer may publish a fee schedule, but allow providers and beneficiaries to negotiate the actual price of the goods or services exchanged. The beneficiary is free to accept a higher price while the provider is allowed to go lower. Under such circumstances, the reasonable market price for that particular good or service will be defined at the exchange, and the beneficiary will be placed at the forefront of the negotiating effort. Moneys agreed to beyond the listed fee schedule are borne by the consumer. Moneys saved over the listed fee will be split between the consumer and the payer. In this way, the consumer always has an interest in seeking cost containments even beyond the recommended fee schedule.

The expansion of HSAs and elimination of mandatory fee schedules would make closed provider networks largely obsolete. Presently, health insurance companies rely on provider networks to compete for enrollees. These are groups of providers selected and contracted by the third-party payer as an exclusive group of individuals and organizations at deep discounts to the insurer. The participating provider agrees not to charge the patient more than what the plan allows, and in exchange, he or she gains exclusive access to the third-party payer's beneficiaries.

Under this model, the patient and the provider alike are isolated from the effects of the free market . The patient need not negotiate for a satisfactory price from the provider and doesn't even need to know what that price is because the reimbursement has already been negotiated and set by the insurer. The provider too doesn't need to worry about the prices charged for the services rendered since it has been set for her. Just as importantly, the provider likely does not even know how much she is getting paid for a particular procedure. And thus, price transparency disappears.

Through the massive conglomerate of participating providers and beneficiaries, the laws of supply and demand are buffered, and the opportunities for new players to enter the market are thwarted. The result is the concentration of enrollment within the present market participants and the consequent increases in prices.

In 2014, for instance, there were 37 states where the three largest insurers accounted for at least 80% of the total enrollment,[351] and in that same year, in Alabama, Blue Cross and Blue Shield accounted for 97% of the state's enrollees.[352] HSAs, of course, will disrupt this milieu as will the elimination of mandatory fee schedules. Patients will immediately be in the position to price hunt and negotiate just like they do in practically any other portion of the American economy. Providers would immediately become intimately aware of their charges and would be rushing to publish them. The issue of price transparency with which so many policymakers grapple will instantly disappear. And the consumer (patient/beneficiary) would instantly know how much financial support is being offered him or her under his or her insurance plan for his care.

Additionally, since there would be no closed networks, patients could equally access any provider they wished, not just those approved by their payer. No longer would providers be locked into one network or another as they strive to grow their clientele. No longer would new and novel insurers struggle to enter the market because of an inability to access and contract providers. And more importantly, no longer would patients be restricted from being able to see one physician or another based on provider network membership and participation. Instead, the only factors determining whether a patient wishes to be taken care of by a particular provider are the distance traveled to be seen and whether the price is appropriate for the service.

Similarly, government-mandated prices have little place in a system that correctly touts the free market as the most effective method of conducting commercial exchanges. Price limitations create shortages, and shortages in healthcare translate to a shortage of products and services. We have specifically seen the effects in the pharmaceutical industry where Medicare's mandated price limitations are the direct cause of generic, prescription medication, in particular, cancer medications. The government needs to stop reaching for price caps as the answer to expensive medications and acknowledge that it is competition that will control drug prices.

As we noted in Chapter 3, eliminating such market restriction will not only allow for the lowering of drug prices, but will promptly cause many of the over 200 drugs presently in the shortage list to be amply supplied.

A comment is in order here regarding "Any-Willing-Provider Laws" and how they relate to the proposal of doing away with mandatory fee schedules. In an Any-Willing-Provider model, the insurance company is required to pay any provider who is willing to honor the insurer's terms in treating its beneficiaries. Under these legislations, a patient may go to any provider, whether she is in network or not, and ask to be seen under the conditions developed by the insurer. If the non-participating provider voluntarily agrees to see the patient under the insurance company's terms, the insurance would be legally obligated to pay that non-participating provider the same way it pays its participating providers.

Such laws allow for greater choice on the part of the patient and provider alike since they no longer need to commit to an insurance company to accept a patient or contract a provider. On the other hand, the insurer loses whatever leverage it has in obtaining volume discounts from providers. The insurer could also have the government unduly intrude in its contracting rights by forcing it to participate with a provider with whom it would not otherwise work.

Any-Willing-Provider laws are weaker and less conducive to unleashing free market pressures on participants than removing balance billing requirements or HSAs since the insurer still dictates the terms of the interaction; the question is simply whether a provider wishes to accept those terms for any given patient.

The removal of mandated fee schedules works differently in that it would essentially turn the insurer's beneficiaries into an army of negotiators on the part of the insurer, and there would no longer be a need for the insurer to even establish a network. All the costs associated with network recruitment would be gone. The insurer would only need to worry about two things: deciding how much it is willing to pay for a procedure or interaction and publishing that number so that its beneficiaries would know.

Promoting Interstate Insurer Competition and Mobility

Because politicians and policymakers have changed the role of healthcare insurance from risk diverting agreements to payment plans for foreseeable health expenses, health insurance companies have been forced to provide coverage enrollees may not require or desire. For example, the ACA requires small business insurance policies to cover ambulatory patient services, emergency services, hospitalization, maternity and newborn care, mental health and substance use disorder services, prescription drugs, rehabilitative and habilitative devices and services, laboratory services, preventive and wellness services, chronic disease management, and pediatric services.[353] The ACA also prohibits persons over 30 years of age from purchasing catastrophic insurance unless they meet certain exemptions, and requires insurers to cover certain preventive services.[354] Each one of those mandated coverage provisions limits consumer choices and increases premiums.

Suppose a young, male carpenter, in great health, with a family wishes to purchase health insurance. He may either be self-employed or own a small business. He is worried about the possibility of getting injured at work or having a time-limited illness, such as appendicitis, the treatment of which would cost a significant amount and potentially keep him from earning money for several months. He may desire only a catastrophic plan or a plan covering only hospitalizations. Such coverage would be tailored to fit his needs and would be less expensive than a more inclusive plan. Under the ACA, such a plan would not qualify for the health insurance tax break. If he purchased that insurance and that insurance alone, not only would he be on the hook for the coverage he purchased, but he would either have to purchase more insurance until his plan met the regulatory requirements for qualified insurance coverage or he would have to pay the health tax in addition to the insurance premium. As a result, he would likely not purchase a limited coverage plan. Rather, he would pay the extra money for the more comprehensive coverage to qualify for a tax exemption. His attempts at being frugal would have been thwarted, and he would have less money at his disposal for investment or allocations to other areas of his life. Alternatively, he could decide to forego purchasing health insurance, but if he did so, he would have to pay a fee (a tax according to the Supreme Court).

From the insurer's standpoint, when enough clients such as the one just described encounter the same or similar stumbling blocks, the futility of providing such limited coverage becomes obvious. Because government manipulated the market into making certain options economically unfeasible, the insurer will faze out those more limited plans altogether so that they would no longer be available.

But even without the Obamacare restrictions, there is a sea of seemingly endless regulatory requirements that artificially elevate insurance premiums and limit competition within a jurisdiction. In the case of the same young carpenter interested only in catastrophic coverage, his state may have passed legislation requiring that all insurance companies cover mammograms and breast cancer surgery.

But he is a 25-year-old male working a construction job! The chances of him getting breast cancer during the coverage period are beyond remote, you say.

No matter, responds the state. Fifteen percent of all breast cancer cases actually occur in males, and thus forcing him to purchase this extra coverage will benefit the greater good. Besides, the state continues, premiums will increase by only a small amount. Our carpenter wouldn't even notice it.

But there are other effects from the asymmetric application of requirements. The introduction of the myriad of state-specific coverage requirements serves as an impediment to other insurers against entering a new market. Their opportunity for success may be limited due to the added compliance requirements, and the oligopoly continues.

Then there is the medical loss ratio (MLR) restriction. To prevent insurers within a jurisdiction from unnecessarily raising prices beyond an amount acceptable to government, state regulators and the ACA cap the minimum percentage of an insurer's total revenue it spends on direct healthcare expenditures. The ACA, for example, caps the minimum MLS at 80, meaning that at least 80% of an insurance company's premium revenues must be spent in payments to its beneficiaries' actual medical costs. The remaining 20% may be spent on everything else, including administrative costs, infrastructure, and facility expenses, and profits. If the insurer's MLS falls below the prescribed percentage, then its beneficiaries are subject to price rebates to make up for the discrepancy.

Many states had MLR requirements prior to Obamacare, but they tended to be lower, such as 68 percent. Some states even had no MLR restrictions at all. Obviously, higher MLS requirements made it less attractive for insurers to enter a state's market.

Popular as they are in the eyes of statists, MLR restrictions may actually result in the artificial elevation of premiums. Suppose an insurer normally raises $1 million in premiums. Under an MLS requirement of 80, $800,000.00 would have to be used for payment directed to the treatment of medical conditions. The insurer would have 20% of its premiums, or $200,000.00 available for discretionary spending.

Now, suppose the insurance company decided to raise its premiums to collect $1.5 million per year even though it is still only spending $800,000.00 on actual medical expenses. Eighty percent of its premiums would now amount to $1.2 million. Since its healthcare expenditures have not changed, the insurer would be forced to return the difference between the $1.2 million and the $800,000 to the enrollees to bring its ratio back to 80%; a total of $420,000.00.

But after having collected $1.5 million instead of $1 million, the insurer would now be left with $300,000 for discretionary spending, not $200,000! By raising its premiums, even artificially, the insurer managed to increase its discretionary spending inclusive of money available to pay dividends to its stockholders by 50%, or $100,000. It therefore pays for the insurer to hike its premiums even under MLR regulations. And without a robust set of competitors in its market to check its prices, why wouldn't the insurer raise its premiums?

One final deterrent to achieving improved flexibility and competition is the issue of portability. In Chapter 3, we saw how the close association between health insurance coverage and one's employer was the result of a historical accident during World War II. Although this coupling is convenient for the employee, it also ties the worker to his or her job. An employee with multiple medical problems would be less likely to leave his job, even a higher paying one, if it meant losing his coverage.

Once again, HSAs and the removal of mandated payment fees would end this dilemma. The employee would no longer be tied to his job by his healthcare insurance. He or she could easily transition to another job without having to worry about insurance networks or even keeping his or her physician. Additionally, tax policy could be modified so that various types of contributions made by the employer to employee health plans would become tax-deductible, whether they be direct purchases by the employer, subsidies made to the employees individually healthcare insurance plan, or used funding for the employee's HSA. This tax law intervention would go a long way towards ending America's artificial dependence on employer-based health insurance and transition the control of Americans' healthcare plans to the individual.

Solving Our Nation's Healthcare Provider Shortage Problem

The United States is riddled by an undersupply of healthcare providers. The driving force behind this provider shortage is the projected increased demand for physician services from the baby boomers, namely that subsegment of the population born between 1946 and 1964. In 2011, 77 million baby boomers reached age 65.[355] By 2030, the number of baby boomers between the ages of 66 and 84 is expected to hover about 60 million people, only to drop back down to 24 million in 2060, at which time baby boomers will be older than 95 years of age.[356]

The United States is woefully underequipped to take care of this massive volume of high-demand patients. By 2032, the United

States will have a shortage of about 122,2000 physicians.[357] Not only does the undersupply of qualified doctors represent a threat to the overall health of American citizens, but economists correctly predict that it will be a significant cause of increased prices for healthcare services[358] in a nation where medical professionals are already the highest paid in the world.[359]

Policymakers aim to address this shortage by changing medical licensure laws so that non-physicians may be able to practice medicine in an unsupervised manner. Although the quest to expand the productivity and utilization of non-physicians is laudable, when such function is expanded to the point where personnel are engaged in activities they are ill-equipped to handle, the consumer is placed at a substantial risk of harm, and the benefits of their expanded participation in healthcare delivery is outweighed by the danger in which the public is placed.

There is a reason why physicians undergo such exacting and protracted training. The practice of medicine is a dangerous and complicated enterprise that risks the lives, safety, and wellbeing of not only the providers, but more tragically, of the patients themselves. Of course, specially trained personnel such as advanced registered nurse practitioners (ARNPs), and physician assistants (PAs) should, under specific circumstances, be allowed to engage inpatient care while not under the direct, real-time supervision of a physician. But subject to the supervision of a physician, to one capacity or another, they must remain, or we knowingly place innocent Americans in danger of preventable complications and tragic outcomes.

If there are insufficient numbers of physicians then the answer is simply to make more of them! Presently, the United States is graduating 23,435 medical and osteopathic-medicine students each year.[360] In the meantime, the number of first-year residency positions in the

United States is 30,232, exceeding the number of medical graduates by 6,797 *each year*.[361] Amazingly, the United States is presently relying on foreign medical graduates to fill these empty residency slots, but this ignores the problem, which is that we are not training enough of our citizens to become doctors or other healthcare providers. What's more, we are not incentivizing them to seek such training. Many of these newly trained, foreign physicians opt to go back to their native countries to practice medicine, while in the United States, countless young Americans eager to take care of their fellow citizens remain devoid of the training they desire and our dependence on foreign medical graduates unnecessarily increases.

Expanding training opportunities for *American* physicians seems to be the most logical approach to the worsening physician shortage in the United States. Not only will we have a much more capable, highly trained, versatile, and robust provider force in so doing, but it will counteract the alleged price elevation from their undersupply.

ARNPs and PAs can be trained to perform many of the duties traditionally carried out directly by physicians. Today, many assist in surgery; actually performing portions of an operation while the attending surgeon is busy at work on another portion. Some ARNPs and PAs see patients in the office setting, evaluating them, and even developing treatment plans without directly consulting the doctor. These assets represent a massive expansion of the physician footprint and an enhancement of his or her flexibility and adaptability when employed safely and judiciously. But ARNPs and PAs are not physician substitutes. Their training differs significantly from physicians, being briefer and less broad. Without going through the rigorous training afforded by our medical schools and subsequent residency programs, ARNPs and PAs are simply not in the position to independently evaluate and treat the full gamut of medical conditions and to properly address them. Unquestionably, new and innovative ways of employing these valuable members of the healthcare delivery system must be developed and laws implemented to support these innovations, but ultimately an appropriately trained physician must supervise these personnel.

Telemedicine is another resource through which physician productivity and supply may be enhanced. Telemedicine is a product of recent technological advances whereby a physician may practice his or her craft while physically separated from the patient. Through telemedicine, a doctor could take care of a patient on the other side of the world!

There are numerous advantages to telemedicine. The patient benefits from the convenience of being able to access a physician or his substitute nearly 24 hours per day. Patients in remote locations suddenly have access to healthcare professionals where they otherwise would not. Some patients may have a sense of greater privacy or even anonymity when remotely accessing medical services.

But there are also limitations. The information available to the diagnostician in a telemedicine encounter is, by definition, limited. The reliability of the data being obtained from the patient, whether historical or objective, is inferior to in-person interactions. Moreover, certain conditions require tactile information, data points only obtainable only through the laying of hands upon the patient. And of course, telemedicine is less personal. Telemedicine may be a very appropriate and powerful tool for many situations, but grossly inappropriate for others, and the interested promoter of a telemedicine product may not always be the most objective party at identifying the line between the two.

There are administrative and legal considerations to telemedicine as well. Who regulates these remote physicians when one party is present in a different state? As we have previously noted, physician regulation is generally state-centric. Does a telemedicine doctor need to be licensed in all fifty states to remotely access patients or does licensure in one state suffice? If the patient is in one state and the doctor is in another, under whose auspices does the physician practice, the state where he is, or the state where his patient is located? And by the way, under what model should the remote physician be paid? Will the insurer honor remote services or do they come out of the patient's pocket? And if the insurer were to cover those services, would it do so at the same rate as it does in-person services?

How about medical malpractice considerations? The general legal dictum is that the plaintiff in a civil suit may bring a defendant to the jurisdiction where he or she resides, or at the very least, the jurisdiction where the offense took place. Where exactly is that in a telemedicine interaction? The answer to this question would dictate so many other issues. For example, each state has its own requirements regarding the amount of medical malpractice coverage a physician must carry in order to practice. In some states that amount is $250,000.00 per malpractice occurrence and $750,000.00 total occurrences within a finite period (usually a year). In others, no medical malpractice insurance is required if the physician meets certain eligibility criteria. When a physician wishes to practice in a state with different malpractice insurance coverage requirements than in the state where he or she is licensed, with which state's malpractice coverage requirements does that physician need to comply, and is he or she eligible for sanctions for not complying with a certain state's malpractice coverage requirements?

Finally, each physician must be accountable to an overseeing authority like a state licensing board. The issue of identifying which board is important, as is making sure that such a board has jurisdiction over the physician and is sufficiently robust to discipline him as necessary.

Unquestionably, telemedicine has the capacity of going a long way towards increasing each physician's reach with the result of fostering competition and developing market disrupters that will lower the costs of healthcare. But telemedicine cannot be safely deployed without ironing out these administrative, scope, and safety questions.

Fighting the Medical Malpractice Strain on Healthcare

Physicians and other medical personnel must be held accountable for the damages they cause through their irresponsible or reckless actions. However, the effort at seeking justice and compensation for disaffected patients cannot be used to stack the decks against the overwhelming majority of providers who make up the nation's healthcare workforce. The medical malpractice debacle that began in the nineteenth century continues today with an estimated cost of $55.6 billion per year! As a result, about $45.6 billion are unnecessarily spent per year on defensive medicine efforts.[362] Then as now, medical malpractice is driven by opportunistic lawyers supported by physicians eager to raise their status through salacious attacks on their colleagues. The effect is not merely pecuniary as countless youngsters are deterred from even seeking a medical education due to the many stories they have heard regarding the hostile legal environment in which they will practice. Additionally, all over the country, physicians or their insurers are paying upwards of a $100,000.00 to earn the legal right to be able to say, "See, I told you so," to a salivating plaintiff attorney with a lawsuit that is frivolous in all eyes other than the legal profession's.

200

State regulatory efforts at curtailing unnecessary litigation have had mixed results. The late 1990s and early 2000s saw the appearance of various forms of state laws seeking to cap medical malpractice damage awards in the hopes of thwarting medical malpractice actions. Although helpful, many of these laws have been overturned by the judiciary on constitutional grounds. Truly, the goal ought not to be to discourage appropriate suits from proceeding, but only those that are ill based.

There are a couple of targeted solutions that although difficult to enact strike at the heart of the problem and ought to be implemented. The first is the establishment of medical courts. These bodies are made up of medical panels that quickly identify and dispose of meritless cases. The turn around time for these review bodies can be as short as 90 days, and they can offer the opportunity to remove cases from the dockets at savings of scores of thousands of dollars to each of the parties with the added advantage of freeing up the courts for more serious cases. Additionally, physicians who offer misleading or fraudulent testimony ought to be made responsible for the costs incurred by the opposing party to counteract the effects of their testimonies. These two steps alone will go a long way toward ameliorating the horrific legal environment in which our physicians practice today.

Cutting the Costs of Inpatient Care

We have already reviewed the devastating effects of hospital care in the United States upon the total costs of healthcare delivery. These prices have exploded to such an extent, that as noted in Chapter 4, hospital-related expenditures now account for about 32% of the nation's total healthcare expenditures.[363] If we are to cut costs of hospitalizations, then the price controlling forces of the free market must be allowed to function upon these institutions as well. In an environment where facilities are paid a set amount for a hospitalization regardless of the number of services or procedures delivered in support of that hospitalization, allowing physicians to own hospitals and have a stake in the profits and expenses of running the facility makes all the sense in the world. Just as it did with the Health Planning Resources Development Act in 1974 where the government interfered with the market over a perverse interpretation of supply and demand, Congress, through the Affordable Care Act, decided that physician ownership of hospitals was counterproductive to cost controls, thus passing a partial prohibition on physician ownership of hospitals that participate in Medicare and Medicaid.[364] Consequently, about 37 hospitals were never built, and 40 hospital projects remained unfinished simply because of the Obamacare-imposed prohibition on physician ownership of hospitals.[365]

The perverted economic theory behind the prohibition of physician ownership of hospitals is that if doctors were allowed to own hospitals, they would engage in self-referral practices designed to increase income generation for their hospitals, and themselves, at the expense of the patient. What the statist policymakers fail to consider (or chose to ignore) is that hospitals are generally paid a predetermined amount for services. As such, physician ownership of hospitals actually serves as a cost suppressor since they would then share in the interest of cutting costs and not engaging in unnecessary procedures or investigations. What's more, physician-owned hospitals tend to outperform conventional hospitals in value-based assessments.[366] In fact, whereas 40% of physician-owned hospitals receive CMS's 5-star rating, only 5% of non-physician hospitals receive this prestigious quality standard.[367] Once again, Congress errs in ignoring the salutary forces within the free market, choosing instead to ostracize it with predictably negative results.

Curbing the costs of hospitalizations also means ending the disparity in reimbursements between them and outpatient care facilities. There is simply no excuse to pay a hospital an amount different than would be paid to a surgery center for identical procedures. As a whole, hospitals may take care of patients with higher acuities than free-standing facilities, but such adjustments ought to be based on the acuity level of the individual being cared for and not a carte blanche correction that unfairly favors hospitals over other venues of care. Additionally, state assistance for hospitals to support them in the quest of delivering care to a community's indigent population should not be purely based on the revenue lost for services delivered to indigents as reported by the hospital. Doing so encourages these institutions to keep their reimbursement rates artificially elevated knowing that in so doing they will be able to report higher losses to government and enhance their reimbursements from the state.

The GPO anti-kickback exception applicable to hospitals must also be discontinued. As we discussed in Chapter 3, this provision unnecessarily adds $600 billion to the nation's healthcare bill and limits the participation of drug companies with a desire to enter the generic drug market. The anti-kickback exception in the Social Security Act must be repealed so that all entrepreneurs desiring to bring less expensive drugs and medical equipment to the market may do so without being inhibited by a government-created disadvantage to their efforts. Of course, hospitals and other mid-chain consumers will be able to continue using GPOs, but they ought no longer be motivated to do so through under-the-table payments given to them by the very entities with which they are conducting business.

But if cost containment necessarily includes leveling the playing field on reimbursements for hospitalizations, it must also include putting an end to restrictive laws that keep new hospitals from flourishing. CONs must not be required as a prerequisite to a hospital opening its doors, or expanding its services within a community. The premises for such laws are ill-founded and destructive to competition. If a group of investors sees an opportunity to excel in a community, let them pursue it. The competition and increased availability of services will cut prices. If the product is to be a specialty hospital such as a cardiac or cancer center, then encourage its construction. Do not impede it. The model will either work or give way to another, more effective and productive one. Neither MedPAC nor any other government agency ought to be dictating to the private hospital the circumstances under which it should build a stand-alone emergency room. If such a facility is allowed to operate under state law (not all states allow for the operation of a stand-alone emergency room), then the federal government ought to have no role in deciding the conditions under which such a facility ought to be built or operated. See Chapter 5 for details on how MedPAC has manipulated the market to favor the construction and operation of certain stand-alone emergency rooms over others.

Relatedly, the government must stop skewing the models through which healthcare is delivered within a community to give hospitals unfair advantages in the market place, or greater control of it. Favorable reimbursements for ACOs ought to be shunned. If ACOs truly add value, then let them realize their greater profits through cost savings, not through greater reimbursements arbitrarily awarded to them by government. Similarly, bundled payment models ought not be encouraged by government nor prohibited. They should arise naturally...or not.

Arguably the sector where the free market has the greatest potential for beneficial impacts in healthcare is in the area of hospital administration. Hospitals must compete against hospitals for what they do best and other providers must compete against similarly based providers for their business. Only by allowing this equity in competition do we will realize a truly efficient and quality-enhanced healthcare delivery system.

Direct Primary Care, One-Stop Shopping, and Healthcare Ministries

One of the great strengths of the free market is its ability to conjure up ways of radically reconfiguring goods or services to either dramatically improve them or to provide them at significantly lower costs. The automobile, computers, portable communications, and retail sales are examples of markets fundamentally affected by disrupters that served not only to massively expand the production of these goods and services, but also to place them in the hands of countless people who would not otherwise have had access to them. Healthcare is no exception.

In the provider access arena, there is direct primary care (DPC). Born out of concierge medicine, DPC is the concept of accessing your primary care physician directly, unlimitedly, and without interference from third-party payers. Here, the patient enters into an agreement with his primary care provider whereby he may visit the doctor unlimitedly in exchange for a monthly fee. In its infancy, DPC was known as concierge care and accessible only to people of means who were willing to pay top dollar to have a physician at their beck and call. Concierge medicine was a market disruptor in that it allowed a segment of the population to secure access to a physician 24 hours a day without having to deal with long wait times or obtaining approval from their third party payers to access services.

For the physician, concierge medicine was advantageous because it allowed her to simplify her practice, as well as her life. No longer would she have to pay thousands of dollars a year for specialized personnel whose only purpose it is to deal with insurance companies, nor did she have to deal with the administrative challenges needed to procure payment. The patient simply paid a monthly or yearly fee for the service while the physician worried only about collecting the fee and being available to provide the necessary care.

Over time, the market disruptor was itself disrupted. Primary care physicians learned that they could charge lower monthly fees in exchange for offering their services for a larger number of patients, particularly if the physician was able to hire a few market expanders such as nurse practitioners or physician assistants to accommodate the larger number of patients. In time, DPC became so accessible, that in many communities, they were available (and still are) for a mere $50.00 per month.

The major challenge to DPC is its definition. Legally, participants in these arrangements describe their products as club memberships. In exchange for a periodic fee, the patients gain membership to a club the benefits of which include unlimited access to the physician and his staff. The insurance lobby counters by claiming the arrangements are really insurance policies since the monthly payments actually represent insurance premiums to cover the patient for such times when he or she would need to see a doctor, no different from what conventional insurance policies offer today. Most threateningly for DPC, some court rulings have agreed with the legal arguments from the insurance industry. Consequently, some state legislatures have passed laws simply declaring that DPC is not insurance. DPC continues to be a formidable tool through which patients may access care in a less expensive, more convenient manner. Not only does it appear as a conduit of great reform within the medical industry, but also it may supplement other efforts to cut the costs of government-funded care. This model must be fully developed in support of a more streamlined system of accessing care.

Similar to DPC in their power to disrupt the healthcare market are the one-stop shopping arrangements popping up in the surgical sector. Surgical services do fit into a DPC service model because surgery generally is a one-time event, not a recurring one like going to one's primary care physician. Yet many patients have difficulty affording surgery when they are not insured due to the high price of the service. Some centers, such as the Surgery Center of Oklahoma, have developed a payment model to alleviate this strain. According to Dr. Keith Smith, founder of the Center, his colleagues and he have developed a model whereby they offer the patient a single price to cover all services associated with a surgical event, kind of like a bundled payment model, but without the government interference.[368]

Under this model, the patient simply informs the Center of what he needs to have done. The Center quotes him a single price and then finds the surgeon, the anesthesiologist, the pathologist, the radiologist, and the physical therapist, among other goods and services as may be required.

Over the years, the Surgery Center of Oklahoma has developed a network of health professionals willing to work within the prearranged prices collected directly from the patient. According to Dr. Smith, the Center is in a position to offer such disruptive prices because they minimize the facility fee to bare-market levels and increase reimbursements to the people who work at the center such as the surgeons and the anesthesiologists.[369] Amazingly, and in stark contradiction to the report from major economic foundations and various government agencies regarding the price of healthcare, the Surgery Center of Oklahoma has essentially maintained similar or same prices for the past 20 years![xxxv]

The Center then searched for other advantages in offering and delivering its services by enticing employers to refer their outpatient surgical services to them. This allowed the Center to expand its base while solidifying a viable and inexpensive healthcare alternative for employees and further freeing them from the pressure of purchasing healthcare insurance.

Admittedly, these arrangements do not address the cost of a major hospitalization, but such costs may be borne through either self-insurance by the employee or the employer, or through the purchase of a major hospitalization insurance product for pennies on the dollar over what a conventional insurance policy would cost.

Then there are healthcare sharing ministries, like Medi-Share, set up as not-for-profits. Here, people with a common moral calling contribute to a savings account that they manage. These common funds cover the healthcare costs of those contributors who may not otherwise have been able to afford it, and they have been successfully providing this service in a self-sustained manner since the 1990s. Healthcare sharing ministries are becoming increasingly popular as a method for accessing funding for medical expenses without paying the high costs of medical insurance.

Finally, a comment must be made regarding the rarely encountered, but successful, voluntary reimbursement model, or priceless pricing. According to Dr. Venu Julapalli one of the concept's pioneers,

---

[xxxv] Interestingly, this is the same price stability encountered by Dr. Lee Gross in his DPC center, Epiphany Health, in North Port, Florida.

priceless pricing represents "an experiment in outrageous love."[370] Essentially, the physician offers no required prices, only a recommended price list. What the patient pays is purely up to him and based only on the value the patient assigns to the treatment being delivered. Amazingly, the model has been profitable and may fundamentally transform how Americans pay for their healthcare devoid of government or corporate interference.

The Uninsured and Pre-existing Conditions

If we enact these changes the issue of the uninsured and pre-existing conditions in this country. Remember, the uninsured and those with pre-existing conditions exist only because of the flawed system our country presently employs in funding healthcare. Since HSAs follow the patient for their whole lives, they will never be challenged by a pre-existing condition, nor will they ever truly be uninsured. Parents will be incentivized to fund HSAs for their children from a very early age. And with provisions allowing for tax-deductions, inter-vivos transfers, and divisibility there stands to be very few Americans who would have no resources with which to fund their care. Hence there would be few uninsureds, and pre-existing conditions will become a historical defect of an extinct healthcare funding model.

Additionally, with the salutatory effects of competition and market disruptors, even those with limited or no HSA resources would have greater spending power than they encounter in the present world where government, insurers, and disparate reimbursements serve to artificially prop up prices.

But, of course, although better than the present corrupted system, the free market is not a utopia. Nothing is. And for those limited situations, society as a whole would need to step in.

Government's Role in Free Market Healthcare

Despite the efforts at promoting free market enterprises within healthcare, there is a proper role for government in healthcare. Not surprisingly, our colonial and nineteenth-century predecessors identified many of the key functions government should be playing within this silo. Healthcare directly deals with the most precious commodity each and every one of us has; our lives. It is based on a highly complex science with multiple moving parts. It takes extensive knowledge and skill to safely deliver such care, and if it is not done so appropriately, with great skill and judgment, the ones who suffer for its shortcomings are the patients who come to depend on proven and reliable service. America has already seen the consequences of the unfettered, unobstructed participation of the opportunist in the healthcare market. The footprints of quacks, charmers, oil mixers, and potion makers abounded throughout the eighteenth and nineteenth centuries and have no business in being resuscitated.

Today, like in the earliest days of our national experience, it falls upon the states to establish the credentialing requirements needed to engage in the practice of medicine. Establishing these requirements, policing performance, and developing and enforcing minimum proficiency standards continue to be fundamental functions of the various states. Yes, there is an inconvenience in having the various specialties regulated at the state level over the federal government, but the benefits of maintaining this regionalistic approach vastly outweigh the disadvantages not only as they relate to healthcare regulation, but in preserving the present federalist relationship between the states and the national government. Co-ops entered between states for the recognition of a state's credentialing in another is one solution for increasing the healthcare workforce's interstate interchangeability, but these agreements must be voluntarily entered into by the participating states and not forced upon them through fiat by the federal government.

Government participation is also required in the arena of public health. It is the function of state governments to promote the health, safety, morale, and welfare of their constituents. In few areas is this role more palpably applicable than in ensuring the protection of a state's citizens from the spread of communicable diseases. Tracking the frequency of infectious diseases, identifying hazards for their spread, and developing safeguards such as vaccination programs and other infectious disease prevention methods are foundational to the stability of modern societies. We have seen this play out throughout the nation's history with the fights against smallpox, yellow fever, measles, cholera, and influenza, to name a few. The states, and even the colonies, were essential in developing and distributing vaccinations, creating and maintaining safe houses, imposing quarantines when necessary, and ridding communities of the hazards that served as cesspools for disease.

In a free market, federalist healthcare system, the federal government also has a role in infectious disease prevention and containment. Disease vectors do not recognize political lines and traverse them freely. Oftentimes efforts undertaken in one region of the nation prevents the proliferation of the disease in another, saving not only money and valuable resources, but lives as well. Funding these efforts through a centralized distribution center is crucial, and may be properly undertaken by collaborations between state and federal governments.

But notice these government-related activities specifically apply to the control of infectious diseases, conditions caused by viral or bacterial organisms (and sometimes fungi) capable of being passed from one person to the next, or to humans through other vectors. The prevention of lifestyle-related medical conditions is a far different consideration. Yes, many epidemiologists, physicians, economists, political scientists, and politicians advocate for government-mandated or funded prevention efforts related to lifestyle, but this is an overextension of government's role and a set-up for the evisceration of its restraints. Conditions like obesity, diabetes, hypercholesterolemia, hypertension, coronary artery disease, and others, which are multifactorial in their causes and whose incidence and severity are affected by the lifestyle choices people make, are ones against which we must all fight, but giving government the authority to socially engineer our lives so as to restrict these lifestyle decisions represents an unacceptably dangerous expansion of power. The prohibition of 32-ounce sodas, the restrictions of foods available in schools, and the prohibition of alcohol are all examples of situations where the government, in its zeal to lower costs and prevent diseases resulting from lifestyle decisions, has excessively intruded into the lives of individuals.

The response from the epidemiologist and the public health experts is that in enacting these legislative interventions lives are being saved. But this is an argument without end. Practically any legislative restriction, be it a prohibition on the use of cars, on carrying guns, on using knives, on striking a match, on jaywalking, or on staying out past midnight can save lives. Taken to its logical end, the *parens patriea* role of government will expand to such an extent as to create a dictatorial system of government implemented "for our own good." In the meantime, our humanity is stripped from us and our freedoms are dissolved.

Some speak of government's successful role in curtailing the use of cigarettes and the countless lives such efforts have saved. But the association between lung cancer and cigarette smoking differs in one important way from the other lifestyle-related diseases we have previously considered. Smoking was a single identifiable activity that was the primary cause of a horrible and often incurable disease. It was never one of many factors. Just like illegal opioids with overdose deaths and cocaine use and a myriad of addiction-related disorders, there is a single identifiable cause with consequences so horrid that the deaths of thousands, even millions, ensue. Such is not the case with lasagna, or soft drinks, or butter. As protectors of our liberties and guardians against the undue expansion of government authority, we must remain ever vigilant of possible conduits to the destruction of the delicate balance between the authority of government and our freedoms. Failure to do so will have consequences far greater in magnitude than recklessly reaching for yet another slice of pizza.

There is another role of government that has not yet been explored, but may serve as an appropriate one for it, that of needs-identification. Government, particularly the federal government, is in an enhanced position to quickly identify the foreseeable healthcare needs of a vulnerable population. Through the work of agencies like the CDC, the federal government can identify upcoming threats or challenges to the nation's health earlier than the market or private enterprise may be able to do. Examples where this has happened include threats from diseases like Ebola, the human immunodeficiency virus, certain cancers, opioid dependence, and mental health issues, among others. The federal government is therefore in a position to direct or steer research and development in those areas. Although such research and development should be undertaken by the private sector, government may be able to herald its necessity, particularly in light of upcoming threats, and even provide incentives and funding for such projects. The federal government could therefore fill a large void in our nation's ability to respond rapidly and effectively to developing healthcare threats and even in the effort of averting them. Those needs must be routinely and recurrently scoured so that threats that have already been addressed, or their market become self-sufficient, may be removed from the government's priorities list to make room for the next set of foreseeable threats or challenges.

The topic of threat-readiness is intimately related to the issue of drugs and pharmaceuticals in our country. The FDA, the agency assigned to deal with the nation's drug development, is woefully private sector dependent. As noted in Chapter 3, the FDA is only an approval agency for requests dealing with proposed medications. It possesses no steering mechanism towards the production of medications to deal with the nation's medical afflictions. What's more, the nation's research and development process is patent dependent, meaning that unless a person or organization believes there is a patentable product to be had for their efforts that stands a realistic chance of paying for itself, no one will pursue it. Medical marijuana advocates claim this (along with the Level II designation of marijuana by the FDA) is the chief reason why medical marijuana has not been developed in this country. There is a point to their contention, one that may be solved through the designation of an agency as an overseer of the development of potential medications not deemed to be attractive to market development, but holding the promise of great benefits.

There is also a belief that Medicare and large insurers provide a barrier to the consumer against the exorbitantly high prices of medications. As we have seen, these protections are illusory, brought to us by the fabricated notions created by the same institutions that limit our choices and dissuade competitor entry into the market. In reality, it is because of price regulations imposed by CMS and third-party payers coupled with the suppressive effects of GPOs that such few manufacturers are creating public domain medications. This effect is particularly felt in the arena of intravenous medications, especially in the case of life-sustaining, intravenous, cancer medications.

In a free market system, patent protections could still be in place for seven years as they are now, but the price protections available to the public would be imposed by competition within the market itself. Instead of encountering an exorbitantly elevated price for patented medical products followed by its precipitous price drop once the patent expires, prices would drop through the pressures of supply and demand once a medication entered the post-patent market. The price post-patent manufacturers would charge for their products would likely be similar to what is presently encountered, but the choices and quantity of medicines available to the consumer and for the treatment of medical conditions would be much greater, thus allowing our healthcare system to markedly improve.

One final situation where the government properly provides a role is in risk pool development and funding. There will always exist a segment of the population, either because of circumstance, their medical conditions, disability, or the sheer enormity of the cost of treatment that will be unable to pay for its care. For these rare but important circumstances, government must be prepared to act. For one, government must provide incentives to individuals and organizations willing to charitably fund the care of others. This action of selfless contributions to others is a staple for the nation's foundation and propagation, and ought to be supported by government. Tax incentives for healthcare based charitable organizations, such as health sharing ministries, ought to be maximized. Employers who help fund such participation should be allowed to make contributions on behalf of their employees in a tax-free manner just like they ought to be allowed to contribute to their employees' HSAs.

However, for those few situations where no other path exists, government ought to create high-risk pools that are subsidized by the public at large through tax dollars. Once again, to maximize the benefits of the free market and the protection of our liberties, the footprint of government in this arena should be kept to a minimum; as it stands to be if these free market enhancing regulatory changes are made.

The collective effects of these interventions should be that virtually everyone ought to have the access to the care that has so eluded our nation to this point and has been the subject of such angst throughout our recent national deliberations. A free market approach will also curtail the risk of handing government any more control of our liberties and freedoms than is absolutely necessary. In short, in implementing a free market based system of healthcare delivery, government, be it local, state, or federal ought never be in a position of assessing the value of our lives relative to the care we need, or in determining the healthcare we receive or deserve. In the meantime, that invisible hand identified by Adam Smith will be in a position to guide us in developing the most sensible, efficient, least expensive, and quality loaded methods of delivering care.

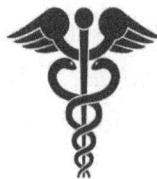

Conclusion

So what's the answer to America's healthcare conundrum?

America's healthcare system must reflect the essence of its foundation and of those principles that served to make the country truly exceptional. First, it must be a system that honors the freedom and independence of the individual as its centerpiece. It must be a system where the primacy of the people over government robustly exists. It must be one in keeping with the constitutional limitations of power placed upon our government by the Framers, and it must lay the decisions regarding one's healthcare squarely upon the patient. Such a system, by necessity, is one based on the free market.

The overarching goal of our legislative efforts as applied to healthcare must be directed at achieving these goals. Over the next few decades, our national effort should be aimed at encouraging and enabling the American people to build their individual HSAs so that they may truly be in control of their care and directly involved in the efforts at price-cutting. Legislation should make it easy for people of all ages to create and build these accounts while giving them the ability to will the remainder to their heirs. The tax-deductible opportunities to build these accounts should be decoupled from any other insurance products, including high deductible healthcare plans, or even public healthcare plans. Everyone, not just members of certain age groups should be offered the opportunity to benefit from the tax deductibility benefits of taking responsibility for their care. Given time, this resource will grow to such an extent that Americans will naturally move away from either a government or a third-party payer funded system, even our nation's seniors.

Of course, there will still be a role for insurance-funded care, but it will be primarily for larger expenses, such as in cases of catastrophic events. Specifically, the nation's reliance on insurance companies will be a thing of the past as Americans learn that they can once again afford their care independently and manage it. Government funding will still be required, but it will be restricted, as the number of people requiring public assistance in funding services disappears. Additionally, by identifying impending health threats to the American people, foreseeing upcoming manufacturing risks, and leading the way in the nation's preventive healthcare policies as they relate to communicable diseases, the government will still play a vital role in ensuring the nation's healthcare readiness.

On the provider side, regulations must be adapted in an effort to support those innovative market disrupters enabling them to do more with fewer resources and lower costs. Legislative hurdles to market disruptors must be removed. Innovations such a healthcare sharing funds, direct primary care, ambulatory care centers, expanded use of nurse practitioners and physicians assistants, one-stop shopping, telemedicine, interstate co-ops, and priceless pricing must be supported so that these cost inhibiting alternatives may be allowed to flourish. Similarly, third-party payers ought to be given the flexibility they need to devise and develop more affordable plans made to fit the increasingly streamlined needs of the consumers.

The nation's Framers did arrive at a system of government through which men and women could climb to heights never before imagined regardless of their backgrounds. This framework is just as applicable to healthcare as it is to any other aspect of our society. All we need to do is let it lead the way.

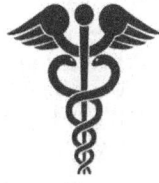

Citations

1 Martha K. Robinson, "Medicine (Colonial Era)," *The Encyclopedia of Greater Philadelphia* (blog), accessed May 25, 2019, https://philadelphiaencyclopedia.org/archive/medicine-colonial-era/.

2 John Russell Twiss, "Medical Practice in Colonial America," *Bull. N. Y. Acad. Med.*, Vol. 36, No. 8, Aug. (1960), 538-539.

3 Robinson. "Medicine (Colonial Era)."

4 Wendy E. Parmet, "Public Health Practices In The Colonial And Federalist Periods," *Bioterrorism, Public Health And The Law 801: Health Care Law Seminar Professor Vernellia R. Randall,* U. of Dayton, 2002 accessed Jun 3, 2019, https://academic.udayton.edu/health/syllabi/Bioterrorism/4PHealthLaw/PHLaw00c.htm.

5 Russell Twiss, "Medical Practice in Colonial America," 538-539.

6 Ibid.

7 Ibid.

8 Robinson. "Medicine (Colonial Era)."

9 Russell-Twiss, "Medical Practice in Colonial America," 542.

10 Robinson. "Medicine (Colonial Era)."

11 Russell Twiss, "Medical Practice in Colonial America," 542.

12 Parmet, "Public Health Practices In The Colonial And Federalist Periods."

13 Ibid.

14 Ibid.

15 Ibid.

16 Cary P, Gross and Kent A Sepkowitz, "The Myth of the Medical Breakthrough: Smallpox, Vaccination, and Jenner Reconsidered," *International Journ. Infectious Dis.*, Vol. 3, No. 1, Jul.-Sept. 1998, 54-60, 55, accessed on Jun. 5, 2019, https://www.ijidonline.com/article/S1201-9712(98)90096-0/pdf.

17 S tefan Riedel, "Edward Jenner And The History of Smallpox And Vaccination," *Proc. Bayl. Univ. Medc. Cent.*, Vol. 18, No. 1, Jan. 2005, 21-25, accessed Jun. 5, 2019 https://www.ncbi.nlm.nih.gov/pmc/articles/PMC1200696/.

18 Riedel, "Edward Jenner And The History of Smallpox And Vaccination.

19 Samuel Bayard Woodward, "The Story of Smallpox in Massachusetts," Annual Oration, Massachusetts Medical Society, 1932, *Massachusetts Medical Society* (blog), Nov. 14, 2016, accessed Jun. 5, 2019, http://www.massmed.org/About/MMS-Leadership/History/The-Story-of-Smallpox-in-Massachusetts/#.XPeY9C2ZORs.

20 Jonathan E. Henry, "Experience in Massachusetts And A Few Other Places With Smallpox and Vaccination," N.E. J. M., Vol. 185, No. 8, 1921. 221-228, accessed on Jun. 5, 2019, https://www.nejm.org/doi/pdf/10.1056/NEJM192108251850802.

21 Ibid.

22 Robinson. "Medicine (Colonial Era)."

23 Parmet, "Public Health Practices in The Colonial And Federalist Periods."

24 Ibid.

25 Gross and Sepkowitz, "The Myth of the Medical Breakthrough," 55.

26 Parmet, "Public Health Practices In The Colonial And Federalist Periods."

27 Ibid.

28 Ann M. Becker, "Smallpox in Washington's Army: Strategic Implications of the Disease During the American Revolutionary War," Journ, Mil. Hist, Vol. 68 April 2004, 381-430.

29 Ibid.

30 Ibid.

31 Ibid.

32 Ibid.

33 Russell Twiss, "Medical Practice in Colonial America," 542.

34 Ibid.,543.

35 Ibid.

36 Parmet, "Public Health Practices In The Colonial And Federalist Periods."

37 United States v. Butler, 297 U.S. 1 (1936).

38 Ryan C. Squire, "Effectuating Principles of Federalism: Reevaluating the Federal Spending Power as the Great Tenth Amendment Loophole." Pepperdine Law Review, vol. 25, issue. 4 (May 15, 1998): 896-898.

39 Nat'l Fed'n of Indep. Bus. v. Sebelius, 567 U.S. ___ (2012).

40 Gibbons v. Ogden, 22 U.S. 1 (1824).

41 Ibid., 195.

42 Ibid.

43 Filburn 317 U.S. 111, at 125.

44 Charles M. Hubbard, "Lincoln and the Chicken Bone Case," American History. Vol. 32. Oct. 1997, 31-34.

45 Allen D. Spiegel, "Defense Lawyer, A. Lincoln Uses Chicken Bones in a Malpractice Case," In A. Lincoln Esquire, A Shrewd, Sophisticated Lawyer in his Time (Mercer University Press 2002): 116-140.

46 Jacob R. Freese, Dep. Aug. 11, 1857.

47 Ibid.

48 Hubbard, "Lincoln and the Chicken Bone Case."

49 Spiegel, "Defense Lawyer, A. Lincoln Uses Chicken Bones in a Malpractice Case."

50 Freese, Dep.

51 Ibid.

52 Ibid.

53 Spiegel, "Defense Lawyer, A. Lincoln Uses Chicken Bones in a Malpractice Case."

54 Ibid.

55 Hubbard, "Lincoln and the Chicken Bone Case."

56 Spiegel, "Defense Lawyer, A. Lincoln Uses Chicken Bones in a Malpractice Case."

57 Robert. L. McLaurin, "Abraham Lincoln's Malpractice Experience," in *A Brief History of Medical Malpractice 2000 B.C. to 2000 A.D.*, 47-52.

58 Hubbard, "Lincoln and the Chicken Bone Case."

59 Spiegel, "Defense Lawyer, A. Lincoln Uses Chicken Bones in a Malpractice Case."

60 Hubbard, "Lincoln and the Chicken Bone Case."

61 McLaurin, "Abraham Lincoln's Malpractice Experience."

62 Spiegel, "Defense Lawyer, A. Lincoln Uses Chicken Bones in a Malpractice Case."

63 McLaurin, "Abraham Lincoln's Malpractice Experience."

64 Spiegel, "Defense Lawyer, A. Lincoln Uses Chicken Bones in a Malpractice Case."

65 Ibid.

66 Ibid.

67 "This Day In History July 30, 1965, President Lyndon B. Johnson Signs Medicare Bill," Truman Library And Museum website, accessed Jun. 10, 2019, https//www.trumanlibrary.org/anniversaries/medicarebill.htm.

68 Julio Gonzalez, *Health Care Reform: The Truth* (Venice, FL: Aragon Publishers, Inc, 2008), 29.

69 Ibid.

70 Howard Markel, "How Medicare Came to Be Thanks to Harry S. Truman," PBS (blog), accessed Jun. 10, 2019, https://www.pbs.org/newshour/health/president-johnson-signs-medicare-law.

71 "Reflections on Implementing Medicare." Restructuring Medicare For The Long Term Project. National Association of Social Insurance website. Jan, 2001, 35, accessed Jun. 10, 2019, https://www. nasi.org/usr_doc/med_report_reflections.pdf.

72 Ibid., 35.

73 "Milestones 1937-2015," Centers for Medicare and Medicaid Services. Jul, 2015, accessed Jun. 10, 2019, https:www.cms.gov/About-CMS/Agency-Information/History/Downloads/Medicare-and-Medicaid-Milestones-1937-2015.pdf.

74 Ibid.

75 Ibid.

76 "Income, Poverty, And Health Insurance Coverage in The United States: 2017," *Newsroom* (blog), accessed Jun. 10, 2019, http://www. census.gov/newsroom/press-releases/2018/income-poverty.html.

77 "HHS FY 2017 Budget In Brief-CMS-Medicare," HHS.gov, accessed Jun. 10, 2019, https://www. hhs.gov/about/budget/fy2017/budget-in-brief/cms/medicare/index.html#f1.

78 Cindy Mann, Director Center for Medicaid and CHIP Services. Memo to Melania Bella, Director Medicare-Medicaid Coordination Office, "Billing For Services Provided To qualified Medicare Beneficiaries (QMBs)," Department of Health and Human Services, Jan. 6, 2012, accessed Jun. 11, 2019, https://www.medicaid.gov/Federal-Policy-Guidance/downloads/CIB-01-06-12.pdf.

79 Robert Pearl, "Major Inflation Would Devastate Healthcare Providers, Payers And, Ultimately, Patients," Forbes (blog), Feb. 27, 2018, accessed Jun. 13, 2019. https://www. forbes.com/sites/robertpearl/2018/02/27/inflation-healthcare/#db81d3d32a63.

80 CPI Inflation Calculator, accessed on June 13, 2019, http://www.in2013dollars.com/us/inflation/1997?amount=100.

81 Joseph R, Antos and James C. Capretta, "ObamaCare's Failed Cost Controls," WSJ (blog), Dec. 20, 2017, accessed Jun. 13, 2019, https://www. wsj.com/articles/obamacares-failed-cost-controls-1513812078.

82 Pearl, "Major Inflation Would Devastate Healthcare Providers, Payers And, Ultimately, Patients.

83 Ibid.

84 Ibid.

85 "Medicaid to Medicare Fee Index," Kaiser Family Foundation (blog) accessed Jun 15, 2019, http://www. .kff.org/medicaid/state-indicator/medicaid-to-medicare-fee-index/?currentTimeframe=0&sortModel=%7B"colId":"Location","sort":"asc"%7D.

86 Ibid.

87 "2017 Physician Workforce Annual Report," Florida Department of Health, Nov. 2017, Fig. 14. accessed Jun. 15, 2019, www.floridahealth.gov/provider-and-partner-resources/community-health-workers/physician-workforce-development-and-recruitment/2017-doh-physician-workforce-report.pdf

88 Ibid., Fig. 13.

89 Ibid., Fig. 15.

90 Ibid.

91 Lee H. Little. "Physicians Continue In Trend of Medicare Opt Outs," *Healthcare Law Blog Preventive Medicine for Your Healthcare Business* (blog), Feb. 4, 2016, accessed Jun. 11, 2019, https://www. healthcarelaw-blog.com/physicians-continue-trend-medicare-opt-outs/.

92 Ibid., Fig. 14.

93 Michael E. Gluck and Richard Sorian, "Administrative Challenges in Managing the Medicare Program," AARP Public Policy Institute, Dec. 2004, 7.

94 Ibid., 6-7.

95 "Public Health and Promoting Interoperability Programs (formerly, known as Electronic Health Record Meaningful Use)," Center for Disease Control, Jan. 18, 2018, accessed Jun. 25, 2019, https://www.cdc.gov/ehrmeaningfuluse/introduction.html.

96 Ibid.

97 Ibid.

98 Ibid.

99 "Medicare National Coverage Determinations Manual," CMS.gov, Ch. 1, Pt. q §§10-80.12 Coverage Determinations, Rev. Feb. 15, 2019, accessed Jun. 25, 2019, https://www.cms.gov/Regulations-and-Guidance/Guidance/Manuals/Downloads/ncd103c1_Part1.pdf

100 *Home Health Care*, Inc. v. Heckler, 717 F.2d 587 (D.C. Cir., 1983).

101 42 C.F. R. §412.3(e)(1) (Oct. 1, 2013).

102 Memo of Decision, *Alexander v. Azar*, No. 3:11-cv-1703, (MPS), p. 25 (USDC CN Mar. 27, 2019).

103 *Id*. 3.

104 42 C.F.R. §419.22(n) (2018).

105 2018 OPPS data Addendum E.

106 Virgil Dickson, "Fear of Denial Could Be Pushing More Joint Procedure Into Outpatient Setting," Modern Healthcare (blog), Oct. 18, 2018, accessed Jun. 27, 2019, https://www. .modernhealthcare.com/article/20181018/NEWS/181019881/fear-of-denials-could-be-pushing-more-joint-procedures-into-outpatient-setting.

107 Peter J. Ferrara, "Saving Money But Costing Lives: The Obamacare Death Panel Should Be Killed Before It's Too Late," *The Washington Times* (blog), Jun. 14, 2017, accessed May 27, 2019, https://www. washingtontimes.com/news/2017/jun/14/obamacare-death-pan-els-should-be-ended/.

108 "Repeal IPAB," *National Review* (blog), Jun. 16, 2011, accessed Jun. 30, 2019, https://www. nationalreview.com/2011/06/re-peal-ipab-editors/.

109 Caitlin Owens, "House Votes To Repeal Another Piece of Obamacare." The Atlantic. Jun. 23, 2015, accessed May 27, 2019, https://www. theatlantic.com/politics/archive/2015/06/house-votes-to-repeal-another-piece-of-obamacare/452064/.

110 "2015 Agency Legislative Bill Analysis, SB 7044," Florida Agency for Health Care Administration, March 12, 2015, 4.

111 Walter R. Hsiang,, Adam Lukasiewicz, et al. "Medicaid Patients Have Greater Difficulty Scheduling Health Care Appointments Compared With Private Insurance Patients: A Meta-Analysis," *Inquiry* Vol. 56: 1-9, Feb. 2019.

112 Ibid.

113 "2017 Physician Workforce Annual Report," Fig. 14.

114 Hsiang, "Medicaid Patients Have Greater Difficulty Scheduling Health Care Appointments Compared With Private Insurance Pa-tients."

115 Daniel H. et al. "The Influence of Medical Insurance on Patient Ac-cess to Orthopaedic Surgery Sports Medicine Appointments Under the Affordable Care Act." *Orthopaedic Journal of Sports Medicine*, vol. 5, 7 Jul. 2017, doi:10.1177/2325967117714140.

116 Veir Seo, Travis P. Baggett., et al., "Access To Care Among Medicaid And Uninsured Patients in Community Health Centers After The Affordable Care Act, *BMC Health Services Research*, vol. 19:291 (2019), accessed May 8, 2019, https://doi.org/10.1186/s12913-019-4124-z.

117 Katherine Baicker, Sarag L. Tauhman, et al., "The Oregon Experi-ment-Effects of Medicaid on Clinical Outcomes," *N. Engl. J. Med.*; Vol. 368 No. 18. pp. 1713-122, May 2, 2013. doi:10.1056/NEJM-sa1212321.

118 Ibid.

119 Damien J. LaPar and Castigliano M. Bhamidipati, "Primary Payer Affects Mortality for Major Operations," *Ann. Surg.* Vol. 252, no. 3, 554-551. Sept. 2010, doi: 10.1097/SLA.0b013e3181e8fd75.

120 Ibid.

121 Stephen Mihm, "How U.S. Health Care Was Built by a Series of Accidents," *Bloomberg* blog), Feb. 24, 2017, accessed May 27, 2019, https://www.bloomberg.com/opinion/articles/2017-02-24/how-u-s-health-care-was-built-by-a-series-of-accidents.

122 Ibid.

123 Ibid.

124 *Musto v. American General Corp.*, 861 F.2d 897 (6th Cir. 1988).

125 Timothy Stoltzfus Jost, "Loopholes in the Affordable Care Act: Regulatory Gaps and Border Crossing Techniques and How to Address Them," 5 St. Louis U.J. Health L. & Pol'y 27 (2011).

126 Ibid.

127 Lori Rittman Clark, "Health Care Reform What Employers Need to Know," *DRI; The Voice of the Defense Bar* (blog), Jun., 2011.

128 Ibid.

129 "Joe the Plumber Becomes Focus of Debate," AP video Oct. 16, 2008, ac cessed Jul. 13, 2019, https://www. bing.com/videos/search?q=spread+the+wealth+obama&&view=detail&mid=F28380C48BB59493A9B7F28380C48B-B59493A9B7&&FORM=VDRVRV.

130 Clark, "Health Care Reform What Employers Need to Know."

131 "Key Facts about the Uninsured Population." Dec. 7, 2018, ac cessed on Jul. 13, 2019, https://www. kff.org/uninsured/fact-sheet/key-facts-about-the-uninsured-population/.

132 Namrata Uberoir, Finegold, Kenneth, et al., "Health Insurance Coverage and the Affordable Care Act, 2010-2016, ASPE Issue Brief," HHS, 2, accessed Jul. 13, 2019, https:// aspe.hhs.gov/system/files/pdf/187551/ACA2010-2016.pdf.

133 John Greenberg, "Medicaid Expansion Drove Health Insurance Coverage under Health Law." *Politifact* (blog), Jan. 15, 2017, accessed Jul. 13 2019, https://www. .politifact.com/truth-o-meter/statements/2017/jan/15/rand-paul/medicaid-expansion-drove-health-insurance-coverage/.

134 Uberoir, "Health Insurance Coverage and the Affordable Care Act."

135 Ibid.

136 *Nat'l Fed'n of Indep. Bus.*, 567 U.S. ___ (2012).

137 Antonin Scalia, dissenting, *Nat'l Fed'n of Indep. Bus. v. Sebelius*, 567 U.S. ___ (2012). pg. 3.

138 Liz Goodwin, "Supreme Court Upholds Obamacare Mandate as a Tax," Yahoo! News (blog), Jun. 28, 2019, accessed Nov. 6, 2019, https://www. yahoo.com/news/blogs/ticket/supreme-court-issue-obamacare-deci-sion-135554880.html.

139 John Roberts, *Nat'l Fed'n of Indep. Bus. v. Sebelius*, 567 U.S. ___ (2012). pg. 32.

140 Scalia, dissenting, *Nat'l Fed'n of Indep. Bus. v. Sebelius*, 4.

141 *Id.*

142 *Id.*, 18.

143 *Id.*, 18.

144 T*exas v. United States of America*, Civ. Act. No. 4:18-cv-00167-O (USDS ND Texas, Dec. 14, 2018), accessed Jun. 1, 2019, https://www.documentcloud. org/documents/5629711-Texas-v-US-Partial-Summary-Judgment.html.

145 Ronald Hamowy, "Medical Disasters and the Growth of the FDA," *Independent Policy Report*, The Independent Institute, February, 2010, 3, accessed Jul. 17, 2019, http://www.independent.org/pdf/policy_reports/2010-02-10-fda.pdf accessed.

146 "Milestones of Drug Regulation in the United States," FDA, accessed Jul. 17, 2019, https://www.fda.gov/media/109482/download.

147 Hamowy, "Medical Disasters and the Growth of the FDA," 5-6.

148 Ibid., 7.

149 Ibid.

150 Ibid., 6.

151 21 U.S.C. 321, §201(g)(1)

152 "HHS FY 2018 Budget in Brief-FDA," HHS.gov, accessed Jul. 14, 2019, https:// www. hhs.gov/about/budget/fy2018/budget-in-brief/fda/index.html.

153 Hamowy, , "Medical Disasters and the Growth of the FDA," 2.

154 "The FDA's Drug Review Process: Ensuring Drugs Are Safe and Effective," FDA, accessed Jul. 18, 2019, https://www.fda.gov/drugs/drug-information-consumers/fdas-drug-review-process-ensuring-drugs-are-safe-and-effective.

155 Yeygenly Feyman, "Reforming the FDA Can Save $900 Million Annually and Generate $4 Trillion in Annual Social Value." Forbes (blog), Executive Summary Apr. 28, 2014, accessed Jul. 14, 2019, https://www.forbes.com/ sites/theapothecary/2014/04/28/reforming-the-fda-can-save-900-million-annually-and-generate-4-trillion-in-annual-social-value/#7e02a294bf94.

156 Ibid., 3.

157 Ibid.

158 Ibid.

159 Ibid., 4-5.

160 Alexander Tabarrok, Chistopher-Paul Mine, and Joseph DiMais, "An FDA Report Card: Wide Variance in Performance Found Among Agency's Drug Review," Manhattan Institute, Apr. 23, 2014, accessed July 14, 2019, file:/// Users/owner2/Desktop/Library/Healthcare/FDA%20Report%20Card%20 Manhattan%20Institute.pdf.

161 Ibid.

162 Ibid.

163 Ibid.

164 "Drug Shortages List," American Society of Health-System of Pharmacists, accessed July 8, 2019, https://www.ashp.org/drug-shortages/current-short-ages/drug-shortages-list?page=CurrentShortages.

165 United States House of Representatives Committee on Oversight And Government Reform, "FDA's Contribution to the Drug Shortage Crisis," 7, Jun 15, 2012.

166 Ibid., 11.

167 Ibid.

168 Ibid., 11-12.

169 Ibid., 4.

170 Statement for the Record by Marjorie Kanof Director, Health Care Clinical and Military Health Care Issues, General Accounting Office. "Group Purchasing Organizations Use of Contracting Processes and Strategies to Award Contract for Medical-Surgical Products," 6, July 16, 2003.

171 United States Government Accountability Office, "Group Purchasing Organizations, Funding Structure Has Potential Implications for Medicare Costs," Fig. 1, Oct. 2014

172 Ibid., 17.

173 Avik Roy, "Reflection on Medicare's 45ht Birthday." *Forbes* (blog), Jul. 1, 2011, accessed Sept. 17, 2019, https://www.forbes.com/sites/aroy/2011/07/01/reflections-on-medicares-45th-birthday/#-307470ca5624.

174 Ibid.

175 Ibid.

176 David Whelan, "Doctors Versus the AMA," *Forbes* (blog), Aug. 17, 2009, accessed Sept. 17, 2019, https://www.forbes.com/2009/08/17/obamacare-doctors-ama-business-healthcare-obamacare.html#371dc5a770d0.

177 *Graduate Medical Education That Meets the Nation's Health Needs*, Committee on the Governance and Financing of Graduate Medical Education, (Washington D.C.: Institute of Medicine of the National Academies, 2014), Table 2-1, accessed Sept. 18, 2019, https://www.nap.edu/read/18754/chapter/2

178 "Total Enrollment at U.S. Medical School and Sex, 2013-2014 through 2017-2018," Table B-1.2, Association of American Medical Colleges, accessed Oct. 19, 2019, https://www.aamc.org/download/321526/data/factstableb1-2.pdf.

179 Table: Preliminary Enrollment Report Fall 2017. American Association of Colleges of Osteopathic Medicine, accessed Oct. 19, 2019, www.aacom.org/docs/default-source/data-and-trends/2017_fall_enrollment_report.pdf.

180 "Liaison Committee on Medical Education," Association of American Medical Colleges, accessed Sept. 18, 2019, https://www.aamc.org/members/osr/committees/48814/reports_lcme.html.

181 Ibid.

182 Ibid.

183 "Reforming America's Healthcare System through Choice and Competition," U.S. Department of Health and Human Services, U.S. Department of the Treasury, U.S. Department of Labor, Dec. 3, 2018, 45, https://www.hhs.gov/sites/default/files/Reforming-Americas-Healthcare-System-Through-Choice-and-Competition.pdf.

184 Ibid., Table 1.

185 Committee on the Governance and Financing of Graduate Medical Education. Graduate Medical Education That Meets the Nation's Health Needs. (Washington D.C.: Institute of Medicine of the National Academies, 2014), 1 accessed Sept. 18, 2019, https://www.nap.edu/read/18754/chapter/2

186 "U.S. Breast Cancer Statistics," Breastcancer.org, accessed Sept. 18, 2019, https://journalofethics.ama-assn.org/article/medical-ethics-and-media-value-story/2014-05.

187 William J. Gradishar, "USPSTF Breast Cancer Screening Recommendations Remain Unchanged Despite Controversy," *Healio* (blog), Jan. 11, 2016, accessed Sept. 21, 2019, https://www.healio.com/hematology-oncology/breast-cancer/news/online/%7B4e79de36-911d-41ef-bed3-3ad171be-2f26%7D/uspstf-breast-cancer-screening-recommendations-remain-unchanged-despite-controversy.

188 "About the USPSTF," U.S. Preventive Services Task Force, accessed Sept. 21, 2019, https://www.uspreventiveservicestaskforce.org/Page/Name/about-the-uspstf.

189 "Section 1. Overview of the U.S. Preventive Services Task Force Structure and Processes," U.S. Preventive Services Task Force, accessed Sept. 21, 2019, https://www.uspreventiveservicestaskforce.org/Page/Name/section-1-overview-of-us-preventive-services-task-force-structure-and-processes.

190 Ibid.

191 "Grade Definitions," U.S. Preventive Services Task Force, accessed Sept. 21, 2019, https://www.uspreventiveservicestaskforce.org/Page/Name/grade-definitions.

192 Ibid.

193 "Archived: Breast Cancer: Screening, 2002," U.S. Preventive Services Task Force, accessed Sept. 21, 2019, https://www.uspreventiveservicestaskforce.org/Page/Document/UpdateSummaryFinal/breast-cancer-screening-2002.

194 "Archived: Breast Cancer: Screening Original Release Date: November 2009," U.S. Preventive Services Task Force, accessed Sept. 21, 2019, https://www.uspreventiveservicestaskforce.org/Page/Document/Update-SummaryFinal/breast-cancer-screening.

195 "Final Recommendation Statement Breast Cancer: Screening," U.S. Preventive Services Task Force, accessed Sept. 21, 2019, https://www.uspreventiveservicestaskforce.org/Page/Document/RecommendationStatementFinal/breast-cancer-screening1#table-of-contents.

196 "Breast Cancer Facts and Figures 2017-2018," American Cancer Society, Table 1, accessed Sept. 21, 2019, https://www.cancer.org/content/dam/cancer-org/research/cancer-facts-and-statistics/breast-cancer-facts-and-figures/breast-cancer-facts-and-figures-2017-2018.pdf.

197 "Risk of Developing Breast Cancer," Breastcancer.org, accessed Jan. 18, 2020, https://www.breastcancer.org/symptoms/understand_bc/risk/understanding.

198 Rachel Roubein, "Preventive Task Force Facing Influx of Lobbying," *The Hill* (blog), Oct. 13, 2016, accessed Sept. 21, 2019, https://thehill.com/policy/healthcare/300922-preventive-task-force-facing-influx-of-lobbying.

199 Peter Wehrwein, "Has the ACA Put the USPSTF in Over Its Head?" *Managed Care* (blog), Nov. 3, 2016, accessed Sept. 21, 2019, https://www.managedcaremag.com/editorsdesk/has-aca-put-uspstf-over-its-head.

200 Roubein, "Preventive Task Force Facing Influx of Lobbying."

201 J. Villani, Q Ngo-Metzger, et al. "Sources of Funding for Research in Evidence Reviews That Inform Recommendations of the US Preventive Services Task Force." JAMA. 2018;319(20):2132–2133. doi:10.1001/jama.2018.5404.

202 "Our Members," U.S. Preventive Services Task Force, accessed Sept. 21, 2019, https://www.uspreventiveservicestaskforce.org/Page/Name/our-members.

203 Ibid.

204 Ibid.

205 Andrew B. Bindman, "JAMA Forum: The Politics of AHRQ," *news@JAMA* (blog), Aug. 3, 2017, accessed Sept. 21, 2019, https://newsatjama.jama.com/2017/08/03/jama-forum-the-politics-of-ahrq/.

206 Pub. L. No. 114-113 § 228 (2015).

207 Thomas Jefferson to William Charles Jarvis, Sept. 28, 1820.

208 J. Mandell, "The Fifth Vital Sign: A Complex Story of Politics and Patient Care," *Clev. Clin. Journ. Med.* 2016 June;83(6):400-401, Accessed Sept. 25, 2019, https://www.mdedge.com/ccjm/article/109138/drug-therapy/fifth-vital-sign-complex-story-politics-and-patient-care.

209 "Quality improvement Guidelines for the Treatment of Acute Pain and Cancer Pain. American Pain Cancer Society Quality of Care Committee," *JAMA*. 1995 dec 20;274(23):1874-80. Accessed Sept. 25, 2019, https://www.ncbi.nlm.nih.gov/pubmed/7500539.

210 JCAHO RI. 1.1.8 quoted in "Joint Commission Changes Its Pain Standards," *Relias Media* (blog), Feb. 1, 2000, accessed Sept. 25, 2019, https://www.reliasmedia.com/articles/44350-joint-commission-changes-its-pain-standards.

211 Ibid.

212 PE. 1.4. Joint Commission on Accreditation of Healthcare Organizations Pain Standards for 2001, Effective January 2001, accessed Sept. 25, 2019, https://www.jointcommission.org/assets/1/6/2001_Pain_Standards.pdf.

213 Ibid.

214 Sonia Moghe, "Opioid History: From 'Wonder Drug' to Abuse Epidemic,'" *CNN* (blog) Oct. 14, 2016, accessed Sept. 25, 2019, https://www.cnn.com/2016/05/12/health/opioid-addiction-history/.

215 Ibid.

216 Claire Felter, "The U.S. Opioid Epidemic," *Council on Foreign Relations* (blog), ForeignAffairs.com, accessed Sept. 26, 2019, https://www.cfr.org/backgrounder/us-opioid-epidemic.

217 Moghe, "Opioid History: From 'Wonder Drug' to Abuse Epidemic.'"

218 Felter, "The U.S. Opioid Epidemic."

219 "Joint Commission Enhances Pain Assessment and Management Requirements for Accredited Hospitals," *The Joint Commission Perspectives* (blog), The Joint Commission, 2017 June;37(7):1. Accessed Sept. 26, 2019, https://www.jointcommission.org/assets/1/18/Joint_Commission_Enhances_Pain_Assessment_and_Management_Requirements_for_Accredited_Hospitals1.PDF; (emphasis added).

220 JCO Standard LD.04.03.13

221 42 U.S.C. §1935.

222 "CON-Certificate of Need State Laws," National Conference of State Legislatures (blog), Feb. 28, 2019, accessed Oct. 21, 2019. http://www.ncsl.org/research/health/con-certificate-of-need-state-laws.aspx.

223 Ibid.

224 "Reforming America's Healthcare System through Choice and Competition," U.S. Department of Health and Human Services, U.S. Department of the Treasury, U.S. Department of Labor, Dec. 3, 2018, 54, https://www.hhs.gov/sites/default/files/Reforming-Americas-Healthcare-System-Through-Choice-and-Competition.pdf.

225 Kacik, "Hospital Price Growth Driving Healthcare Spending."

226 "Reforming America's Healthcare System through Choice and Competition," 54.

227 "CON-Certificate of Need State Laws."

228 "Health Expenditures," National Center for Health Statistics, Centers for Disease Control and Prevention, accessed Jan. 12, 2020, https://www.cdc.gov/nchs/fastats/health-expenditures.htm.

229 Martin Gaynor, Farzad Mostashari, et al., "Making Health Care Markets Work: Competition Policy for Health Care," Apr. 2017, Gaynor, Mostashari & Ginsburg, p. 10-11, https://www.brookings.edu/wp-content/uploads/2017/04/gaynor-et-al-final-report-v11.pdf.

230 Kacik, "Hospital Price Growth Driving Healthcare Spending."

231 Jenny Gold, "Accountable Care Organizations, Explained," Kaiser Health News (blog), Sept. 14, 2015, accessed Oct. 25, 2019, https://khn.org/news/aco-accountable-care-organization-faq/.

232 Eli Cutler, Zeynal Karaca et al., "The effect of Medicare Accountable Organizations on Inpatient Mortality Rates,. Inquiry, 2018 Jan-Dec; 55: published online Set. 24, 2018, accessed Jan. 19, 2020, doi: 10.1177/0046958018800092.

233 "Shared Savings Program: Program Statutes & Regulations," CMS gov, last modified Oct. 1, 2019, accessed Oct. 25, 2019, https://www.cms.gov/Medicare/Medicare-Fee-for-Service-Payment/sharedsavingsprogram/program-statutes-and-regulations.html.

234 Karl Marx, "Critique of the Gotha Program," 1875.

235 "Trans Fat," Food and Drug Administration, accessed Oct. 2, 2019, https://www.fda.gov/food/food-additives-petitions/trans-fat.

236 Laura Donnelly, "NHS Provokes Fury with Indefinite Surgery Ban for Smokers and Obese," The Telegraph (blog), Oct. 17, 2017, accessed Oct. 1, 2019, https://www.telegraph.co.uk/news/2017/10/17/nhs-provokes-fury-indefinite-surgery-ban-smokers-obese.

237 V. Pillutla, H. Maslen, and J Savulescu, "Rationing elective surgery for smokers and obese patients: responsibility or prognosis?" BMC Med Ethics. 2018;19(1):28. Published 2018 Apr 24. doi:10.1186/s12910-018-0272-7.

238 Sibhan Fenton, "Obese People and Smokers 'Banned from Routine Surgery' as NHS Attempts to Cut Spending Cuts," Independent (blog), Sept. 3, 2016, accessed Oct. 2, 2019, https://www.independent.co.uk/life-style/health-and-families/health-news/obese-people-and-smokers-banned-from-routine-surgery-as-nhs-attempts-to-cut-spending-costs-a7223731.html.

239 "National Healthcare Expenditure Data," CMS.gov, last updated Dec. 11, 2018, accessed Oct. 2, 2019, https://www.cms.gov/Research-Statistics-Data-and-Systems/Statistics-Trends-and-Reports/NationalHealthExpendData/NationalHealthAccountsHistorical.html.

240 "How Much Will Medicare for All Cost?" *Health Care* (blog), Committee for a Responsible Federal Budget, Feb. 27, 2019, accessed Sept. 30, 2019, http://www.crfb.org/blogs/how-much-will-medicare-all-cost.

241 Charles Blahouse, Fish J. Charles, Fish, J., and Lillian F. Smith, "The Cost of a National Single-Payer Healthcare System," Mercatus Center George Mason University, July 30, 2018, Table 5, accessed https://www.mercatus.org/publications/government-spending/costs-national-single-payer-healthcare-system.

242 Ibid.

243 Ibid., Table 3.

244 Ibid., Table 5.

245 Elkins, Kathleen, "Here's How Much You Have to Earn to Be in The Top in Every US State," CNBC Make It (blog), Jul. 27, 2018, accessed Oct. 4, 2019. https://www.cnbc.com/2018/07/27/how-much-you-have-to-earn-to-be-in-the-top-1percent-in-every-us-state.html

246 "Options to Finance Medicare for All," Bernie Sanders U.S. Senator for Vermont, accessed Oct. 5, 2019, https://www.sanders.senate.gov/download/options-to-finance-medicare-for-all?inline=file.

247 Nicole Fisher, "Electronic Health Records-Expensive, Disruptive and Here to Stay." *Forbes* (blog), Mar. 18, 2014, accessed July 26, 2019, https://www.forbes.com/sites/nicolefisher/2014/03/18/electronic-health-records-expensive-disruptive-and-here-to-stay/#3934fec65435.

248 "Indiana Medical Records Service Pays $100,000 to Settle HIPAA Breach," HHS.gov, accessed July 26, 2019, https://www.hhs.gov/about/news/2019/05/23/indiana-medical-records-service-pays-100000-to-settle-hipaa-breach.html.

249 Ibid.

250 Jessica Kim Cohen, "Healthcare Data Breaches Reach Record High in April, *Modern Healthcare* (blog), May 10, 2019, accessed July 26, 2019, https://www.modernhealthcare.com/cybersecurity/healthcare-data-breaches-reach-record-high-april.

251 *Sorrell v. IMS Health et al.*, No. 10-779, (U.S. 2011).

252 Latanya Sweeney, "Matching Known Patients to Health Records in Washington State," accessed July 26, 2019, dataprivacylab/projects/wa https://pdfs.semanticscholar.org/e021/e9afdd5c82aeb22102a4140bcfa19f0c49aa.pdf.

253 Dara Kam, "Doctors Win in Florida 'Docs vs. Glocks Legal Tussle." *Orlando Sentinel*, Jun 12, 2017, accessed on July 26, 2019, https://www.orlandosentinel.com/politics/os-docs-vs-glocks-20170612-story.html.

254 Brendan Murphy, "For First Time, Physician Practice Owners Are Not the Majority," AMA, (blog) May 31, 2017, accessed July 29, 2019, https://www.ama-assn.org/practice-management/economics/first-time-physician-practice-owners-are-not-majority.

255 Meg Bryant, "Doctors EHR Frustration Can Influence Patient Satisfaction, Study Finds," Healthcaredive, (blog), May 22, 2018, accessed July 29, 2019, https://www.healthcaredive.com/news/doctors-ehr-frustration-can-influence-patient-satisfaction-study-finds/524032/.

256 Maria Pangioti,, Keith Garaghty, and Judith Johnson, "Association Between Physician Burnout and Patient Safety, Professionalism, and Patient Satisfaction A Systematic Review and Meta-Analyisis," JAMA Network, Sept. 4, 2018. 2018178(10):1317–1331, accessed July 29, 2019, https://jamanetwork.com/journals/jamainternalmedicine/article-abstract/2698144.

257 Ezekiel Emanuel in "Ezekiel Emanuel Confronts Health Care Costs-and Doesn't Like What He Sees." *Penn Medicine News* (blog), Feb. 7, 2013, accessed July 20, 2019, https://www.pennmedicine.org/news/news-blog/2013/february/ezekiel-emanuel-confronts-heal.

258 "National Health Expenditure 2017 Highlights," CMS.gov, accessed July 20, 2019, https://www.cms.gov/Research-Statistics-Data-and-Systems/Statistics-Trends-and-Reports/NationalHealthExpendData/Downloads/highlights.pdf.

259 Ibid.

260 Irence Papanicolas, Liana R. Woski,, and Ashish K. Jha, "Health Care Spending in the United States and Other High-Income Countries," *JAMA*. 2018;319(10):1024–1039, accessed July 23, 2019, doi:10.1001/jama.2018.1150, https://jamanetwork.com/journals/jama/article-abstract/2674671.

261 "The World Health Report 2000 Health Systems: Improving Performance," World Health Organization, 2000, accessed July 23, 2019, https://www.who.int/whr/2000/en/whr00_en.pdf?ua=1.

262 Vivian Ho, Leanne Metcalf, and Cedrick Dark, "Comparing Utilization and Costs of Care in Freestanding Emergency Departments, Hospital Emergency Departments, and Urgent Care Centers," *Ann. Em. Med*. Vol. 70, Issue 6, p, 849, Dec. 2017, accessed Jul. 24, 2019, https://www.annemergmcd.com/article/S0196-0644(16)31522-0/pdf.

263 "National Hospital Ambulatory Medical Care Survey: 2016 Emergency Department Summary Tables," CDC, Table 1, accessed Jul. 20, 2019, https://www.cdc.gov/nchs/data/nhamcs/web_tables/2016_ed_web_tables.pdf.

264 Enard, Kimberly R. and Ganelin, Deborah M., "Reducing preventable emergency department utilization and costs by using community health workers as patient navigators," *Journal of Healthcare Management / American College of Healthcare Executives* vol. 58,6 (2013): 412-27; discussion 428. digital version, 1-2, accessed Jul. 20, 2019, https://www.ncbi.nlm.nih.gov/pmc/articles/PMC4142498/.

265 Ibid.

266 Steven Ross Johnson, "ACA Has Not Reduced ED Visits, Study Finds," *Modern Healthcare*, April 19 2019, accessed Jul. 24, 2019, https://www.modernhealthcare.com/safety-quality/aca-has-not-reduced-ed-visits-study-finds.

267 "National Hospital Ambulatory Medical Care Survey: 2014 Emergency Department Summary Tables," *CDC*. Accessed Jul. 24, 2019, https://www.cdc.gov/nchs/data/nhamcs/web_tables/2014_ed_web_tables.pdf.

268 Baicker, "The Oregon Experiment-Effects of Medicaid on Clinical Outcomes."

269 Steffie Woolhandler, David U. Himmelstein, "The Relationship of Health Insurance and Mortality: Is Lack of Insurance Deadly?" *Ann Intern Med.*, 2017 Sep 19;167(6):424-431. doi: 10.7326/M17-1403. Epub 2017 Jun 27. Accessed Jul. 24, 2019, https://annals.org/aim/fullarticle/2635326/relationship-health-insurance-mortality-lack-insurance-deadly.

270 Ibid.

271 "Raising the Excise Tax on Cigarettes: Effect on Health and the Federal Budget." CBO, iii, Jun., 2012, accessed Jul. 25, 2019, http://www.cbo.gov/sites/default/files/cbofiles/attachments/06-13-Smoking_Reduction.pdf.

272 Jull R. Horwitz, Brenna D. Kelly, and John DiNardo, "Wellness Incentives in the Workplace: Cost Savings through Cost Shifting to Unhealthy Workers," *Health Affairs*, Vol. 32, No. 3 March 2013, accessed Jul. 25, 2019 https://www.healthaffairs.org/doi/full/10.1377/hlthaff.2012.0683.

273 Michael J. McWilliams, Michael E. Chernew, and Bruce E. Landon, "Medicare ACO Program Savings Not Tied to Preventable Hospitalizations or Concentrated Among High-Risk Patients," *Health Affairs*, Vol. 36, No. 12, Dec. 2017, accessed Jul. 25, 2019, https://www.healthaffairs.org/doi/10.1377/hlthaff.2017.0814.

274 Aaron Carroll, "Preventive Care Save Money? Sorry, It's Too Good to Be True," *The New York Times*, (blog) Jan. 29, 2018, accessed Jul. 25, 2019, https://www.nytimes.com/2018/01/29/upshot/preventive-health-care-costs.html?auth=login-email&login=email.

275 "Key Facts About the Uninsured Population" Kaiser Family Foundation (blog), Dec. 7, 2018, accessed Jul. 30, 2019, https://www.kff.org/uninsured/fact-sheet/key-facts-about-the-uninsured-population/#.

276 "Number of nonelderly Adults with Declinable Pre-Existing Conditions under Pre-ACA Practices," Kaiser Family Foundation, accessed Jul. 30, 2019, https://www.kff.org/other/state-indicator/estimated-number-of-non-elderly-adults-with-declinable-pre-existing-conditions-under-pre-aca-practices/?currentTimeframe=0&selectedDistributions=estimated-number-of-nonelderly-adults&sortModel=%7B%22colId%22:%22Location%22,%22sort%22:%22asc%22%7D.

277 "At Risk: Pre-Existing Conditions Could Affect 1 in 2 Americans, or 129 million people," The Center for Consumer Information & Insurance Oversight, CMS, accessed Jul. 30, 2019, https://www.cms.gov/CCIIO/Resources/Forms-Reports-and-Other-Resources/pre-existing.html#_edn1.

278 Henry A. Waxman. and Bart Stupak, "Memorandum: Coverage Denials for Pre-Existing Condition in the Individual Health Insurance Market," Oct. 2010, 1, accessed Jul. 31, 2019, https://oversight.house.gov/sites/democrats.oversight.house.gov/files/documents/Memo-Coverage-Denials-Individual-Market-2010-10-12.pdf.

279 Ibid., 4.

280 "High-Risk Plans Tally Low Uptake Yet Surprisingly Steep Costs," *Managed Healthcare Executive* (blog), May 1, 2012, accessed Nov. 20, 2019, https://www.managedhealthcareexecutive.com/provider-networks/high-risk-plans-tally-low-uptake-yet-surprisingly-steep-costs.

281 Ibid.

282 Kimberly Amadeo, "How Much Did Obamacare Cost?" The Balance (blog), Jun. 25, 2019, accessed Jul. 231, 2019, https://www.thebalance.com/cost-of-obamacare-3306050.

283 "MACRA," CMS, accessed Jul. 31, 2019, https://www.cms.gov/medicare/quality-initiatives-patient-assessment-instruments/value-based-programs/macra-mips-and-apms/macra-mips-and-apms.html.

284 "Federal Subsidies for Health Insurance Coverage for People under Age 65: 2018-2028," Congressional Budget Office, May 2018. 1-2, accessed Jul. 31. 2019, https://www.cbo.gov/system/files/115th-congress-2017-2018/reports/53826-healthinsurancecoverage.pdf.

285 Chuck Dinerstein, "The True Cost of End-of-Life Medical Care," America n Council on Science and Health (blog), Sept. 28, 2018, accessed Aug. 1, 2019, https://www.acsh.org/news/2018/09/28/true-cost-end-life-medical-care-13454.

286 Kelli Whitlock Bruton, "The End of 'Under 12,'" *Pediatrics Nationwide*, Nov. 3, 2014, accessed Aug. 2, 2019, https://pediatricsnationwide.org/2014/11/03/the-end-of-under-12%E2%80%B3/.

287 Chris Welch and Zain Asher, "With Just Weeks Left, Sarah Fights the System for a Life-Saving Pair of Lungs," CNN (blog), May 27, 2013, accessed Aug. 2, 2019, https://www.cnn.com/2013/05/27/health/pennsylvania-girl-lungs/index.html.

288 *Murnaghan v United States Department of Health and Human Services*, Case No. 2:13-cv-03083. June 5, 2013 (ED Penn 2013).

289 Marie McCullough, "A Historic Adult-To-Child Lung Transplant Saver Their Daughter, Who's Now a Thriving Teen," *The Philadelphia Inquirer* (blog), Sept. 10, 2018, accessed Aug. 1, 2019, https://www.inquirer.com/philly/health/sarah-murnaghan-janet-book-adult-to-child-organ-donation-transplant-lungs-philadelphia-hospital-20180910.html.

290 Jay Wolfson, Jay, "A Report to Governor Jeb Bush And The 6th Judicial Circuit in the Matter of Theresa Marie Schiavo," Dec. 1, 2003, 7, accessed Aug. 12, 2019, http://abstractappeal.com/schiavo/WolfsonReport.pdf.

291 Ibid., 8.

292 Ibid., 8-9.

293 Ibid., 9.

294 Ibid., 8-9.

295 Ibid., 12.

296 Ibid., 18.

297 Georg W. Bush. in "A Look Back: The Terri Schiavo Case," CBS News (blog), accessed Aug. 12, 2019, https://www.cbsnews.com/pictures/look-back-in-history-terri-schiavo-death/22/ accessed on Aug. 12, 2019.

298 Spahora Smith, "Charlie Gard Case: American Doctor Arrives Examine Terminally Ill Baby," NBC New (blog) accessed December 19, 2019, https://www.nbcnews.com/news/world/charlie-gard-case-american-doctor-arrives-examine-terminally-ill-baby-n783646.

299 Katie Forster, "Charlie Gard: Parents End Legal Fight to Take Sick Baby to US for Experimental Treatment," *Independent* (blog), Jul. 24, 2017, accessed Aug. 14, 2019, https://www.independent.co.uk/news/uk/home-news/charlie-gard-parents-lawyer-us-end-legal-appeal-us-experimental-treatment-high-court-life-support-a7857431.html.

300 Harley Dixon, "Terminally Ill Boy Denied 'Potentially Life-Saving' Treatment by NHS 'Would Be Given It in Any US Hospital,'" *The Telegraph* (blog) Apr. 3, 2017, accessed Aug. 14, 2019, https://www.telegraph.co.uk/news/2017/04/03/terminally-boy-denied-potentially-life-saving-treatment-nhs/.

301 Debra Goldschmidt and Hilary Clarke, "Baby Charlie Gard Dies after Life Support Withdrawn," CNN (blog), Jul. 28, 2017, accessed Aug. 14, 2019, https://www.cnn.com/2017/07/28/health/charlie-gard-death/index.html.

302 "rationing," *WordNet 3.0*, Farlex clipart collection. S.v., accessed Sept. 5, 2019, https://www.thefreedictionary.com/rationing.

303 "Fraser Institute News Release: One Million Canadians Waited for Medical Treatment in 2017, Costing $1.9 Billion in Lost Wages." Fraser Institute (blog), May 23, 2018, accessed Sept. 8, 2019, https://www.globenewswire.com/news-release/2018/05/23/1510579/0/en/Fraser-Institute-News-Release-One-million-Canadians-waited-for-medical-treatment-in-2017-costing-1-9-billion-in-lost-wages.html.

304 Ibid.

305 Bacchus Barua, "While Politicians Dither, Patients Die," Fraser Institute (blog), accessed Sept. 8, 2019, https://www.fraserinstitute.org/article/while-politicians-dither-patients-die.

306 Scott W. Atlas, "Rationing Healthcare," *Forbes* (blog), Jul. 21, 2009, accessed Nov. 21, 2019, https://www.forbes.com/2009/07/21/rationing-health-care-opinions-contributors-scott-atlas.html#77070a713cb3

307 NHS Constitution for England, § 1, Updated Oct. 2015, accessed Sept. 6, 2019, https://www.gov.uk/government/publications/the-nhs-constitution-for-england/the-nhs-constitution-for-england.

308 Ibid.

309 Ibid., § 4.

310 Ibid.

311 Ibid., Value 6 (p5).

312 Sean Rai-Roche, "CCGs in England Restrict Access to Cataract Surgery," *Optician* (blog), Mar. 3, 2019, accessed Sept. 7, 2019, https://www.opticianonline.net/news/ccgs-restrict-cataract-surgery-in-nhs-england-1.

313 Mike Paulden, "Recent Amendments to NICE's Value-Based Assessment of Health Technologies: Implicitly Inequitable?" *Expert Review of Pharmacoeconomics & Outcomes Research*, Vol. 17: Iss. 3 May 23, 2017, accessed Sept. 6, 2019, https://www.tandfonline.com/doi/full/10.1080/14737167.2017.1330152.

314 "How the UK Rations Health Care," *PRI* (blog), Sept. 17, 2010, accessed, Sept. 9, 2019, https://www.pri.org/stories/2010-12-17/how-uk-rations-health-care.

315 NHS Constitution, § 2.

316 "The NHS Budget and How It Has Changed," The King's Fund, Sept. 5, 2019, accessed Sept. 6, 2019, https://www.kingsfund.org.uk/projects/nhs-in-a-nutshell/nhs-budget.

317 "About MedPAC," MEDPAC, accessed Sept. 11, 2019, http://www.medpac.gov/-about-medpac-.

318 42 U.S.C. § 1395.

319 42 U.S.C. 1395(c)(1)(B).

320 Virgil Dickson, Virgil, "MedPAC Votes to Cut Payments for Free-Standing ERs," *Modern Healthcare* (blog), Apr. 5, 2019, accessed Sept. 12, 2019, https://www.modernhealthcare.com/article/20180405/NEWS/180409947/medpac-votes-to-cut-payments-for-free-standing-ers.

321 "Report to the Congress Medicare and the Health Care Delivery System," MedPAC, Jun. 2018, 58, accessed Sept. 12, 2019, http://www.medpac.gov/docs/default-source/reports/jun18_medpacreporttocongress_sec.pdf?sfvrsn=0.

322 Ibid., 57.

323 Ibid.

324 Ibid.

325 Ibid.

326 Dickson, "MedPAC Votes to Cut Payments for Free-Standing ERs."

327 Steve Blades, "The Back Page: Outpatient Cath Labs Fight for Survival," *Cardiovascular Business* (blog), Sept. 1, 2008, accessed Sept. 13, 2019. https://www.cardiovascularbusiness.com/topics/practice-management/back-page-outpatient-cath-labs-fight-survival.

328 Richard R. Rogoski., "Outpatient Cath Labs Suffer under a System Favoring Hospitals," DAIC (blog), Sept. 17, 2009, accessed Sept. 13, 2019, https://www.dicardiology.com/article/outpatient-cath-labs-suffer-under-system-favoring-hospitals.

329 Blades, "The Back Page: Outpatient Cath Labs Fight for Survival.

330 I bid.

331 "Report to the Congress: Physician-Owned Specialty Hospitals," MedPAC, March 2005, accessed Sept. 13, 2019, http://www.medpac.gov/docs/default-source/reports/Mar05_SpecHospitals.pdf?sfvrsn=0.

332 Ibid., 7.

333 Ibid.

334 Ibid.

335 "The ASC Cost Differential," Ambulatory Surgery Center Association, accessed Sept. 13, 2019, https://www.ascassociation.org/home.

336 Nicole C. Wright, et al., "The recent prevalence of osteoporosis and low bone mass in the United States based on bone mineral density at the femoral neck or lumbar spine," *Journal of Bone and Mineral Research*, vol. 29,11 (2014): 2520-6. accessed Sept 13, 2019, doi:10.1002/jbmr.2269.

337 J.A. Kanis, O. Johnell, et al., "Risk of hip fracture according to the World Health Organization criteria for osteopenia and osteoporosis," *Bone*, Vol. 27; No. 5, Nov. 2000.

338 Kathy Hardy, "Bone Density Testing-Reduced Reimbursement and Access Have Led to Fewer Screening Exams," *Radiology Today*, Vol. 14 No. 10, Oct. 2013, 28, accessed Sept. 16, 2019, https://www.radiologytoday.net/archive/rt1013p28.shtml.

339 Ibid.

340 Peter Steven, "By the Numbers: DXA Testing," National Osteoporosis Foundation, 2018.

341 "Policy Statement: Bone Densitometry Testing," American Alliance of Orthopaedic Executives, 2018.

342 "Medicare: Insolvency Projections," Congressional Research Service, updated Jul. 3, 2019, accessed Oct. 4, 2019, https://fas.org/sgp/crs/misc/RS20946.pdf.

343 *Merriam-Webster OnLine*, "right," accessed Oct. 9, 2019, https://www.merriam-webster.com/.

344 MH Lee, JD Schuur, BK Zink, "Owning the Cost of Emergency Medicine: Beyond 2%," *Ann Emerg Med.* 2013;62(5):498-505, abstract, accessed Oct. 18, 2019, https://www.ncbi.nlm.nih.gov/pubmed/23623558.

345 Table: Health Insurance Coverage of the Total Population, 2017," Kaiser Family Foundation, accessed Oct. 11, 2019, https://www.kff.org/other/state-indicator/total-population/?currentTimeframe=0&sortModel=%7B%22colId%22:%22Location%22,%22sort%22:%22asc%22%7D.

346 Russell Rhine, "Potential for Health Care Savings: Can Health Savings Accounts (HSAs) bend the Cost Curve?" United States Senate Joint Economic Committee, Dec. 13, 2018, https://www.jec.senate.gov/public/_cache/files/baceddcc-39ef-4dae-a216-3da872a738ae/hsa-3.0.pdf.

347 "Health Savings Account (HSA)," HealthCare.gov, accessed Oct. 11, 2019, https://www.healthcare.gov/glossary/health-savings-account-hsa/.

348 Ibid.

349 Amelia M. Haviland, Susan Marquis, et al. "Growth of consumer-directed health plans to one-half of all employer-sponsored insurance could save $57 billion annually." *Health Affairs* (blog) May 2012, accessed Jan 25, 2020, https://www.healthaffairs.org/doi/full/10.1377/hlthaff.2011.0369.

350 Theodore McDowell, "Mandatory Health Savings Accounts and the Need for Consumer-Driven Healthcare, "*The Georgetown Journ. of Law & Pub. Pol.*," 2018 Vol. 16, No pp. 315-337, accessed on Jan. 25, 2020, https://www.law.georgetown.edu/public-policy-journal/wp-content/uploads/sites/23/2018/05/16-1-Mandatory-Health-Savings-Accounts-and-the-Need-for-Consumer-Driven-Health-Care.pdf.

351 "Private Health Insurance: Concentration of Enrollees Among Individual, Small Group, and Large Group Insurers from 2010 through 2013," U.S. Government Accountability Office, Dec. 1, 2014, 4, https://www.gao.gov/assets/670/667245.pdf.

352 Ibid.

353 "Reforming America's Healthcare System through Choice and Competition," fn 264.

354 Ibid., 74.

355 Sandra L. Colby, Jennifer M. Ortman, "The Baby Boom Cohort in the United States 2012 to 2016," United States Census Bureau, May, 2014, 2, accessed Dec. 4, 2019, https://www.census.gov/prod/2014pubs/p25-1141.pdf

356 Ibid.

357 "New Findings Confirm Predictions on Physician Shortage," Association of American Medical Colleges Press Release (blog) Apr. 23, 2019, accessed, Feb. 2, 2020, https://www.aamc.org/news-insights/press-releases/new-findings-confirm-predictions-physician-shortage#.

358 "Reforming America's Healthcare System through Choice and Competition," 30.

359 Ibid., 42.

360 Ibid., 48.

361 Ibid.

362 Rick Ungar, "The True Cost of Medical Malpractice—It May Surprise You," Forbes (blog), Sept. 7, 2010, accessed Jan. 14, 2020, https://www.forbes.com/sites/rickungar/2010/09/07/the-true-cost-of-medical-malpractice-it-may-surprise-you/#7a0b0c042ff5.

363 Kacik, "Hospital Price Growth Driving Healthcare Spending."

364 "Physician Self-Referral: Physician-Owned Hospitals," cms.gov, last modified Aug. 19, 2019, accessed Oct. 26, 2019, https://www.cms.gov/Medicare/ Fraud-and-Abuse/PhysicianSelfReferral/Physician_Owned_Hospitals.html.

365 Kimberly Leonard, "Obamacare Wounds Doctor-Owned Hospitals," *Washington Examiner* (blog), July 10, 2017, accessed Oct. 30, 2019, https:// www.washingtonexaminer.com/obamacare-wounds-doctor-owned-hospitals.

366 AG Ramirez, MC Tracci, et al., "Physician-owned surgical hospitals outperform other hospitals in Medicare value-based purchasing program." *J Am Coll Surg.* 2016 Oct;223(4):559-567, https://www.sciencedirect.com/science/article/pii/S1072751516307207?via%3Dihub

367 "Reforming America's Healthcare System through Choice and Competition," 74.

368 Kevin Smith in "Keith Smith on Free-market Health Care," The Library of Economics and Liberty EconTalk (podcast) Nov. 17, 2019. https://www. econtalk.org/keith-smith-on-free-market-health-care/.

369 Ibid.

370 "Priceless Pricing," ICGmed.com, accessed Dec. 7, 2019, https://igcmed. com/priceless-pricing/.

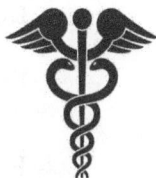

INDEX

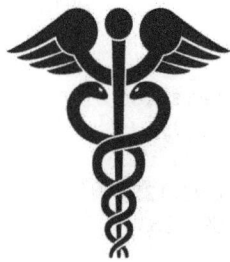

www.ingramcontent.com/pod-product-compliance
Lightning Source LLC
Chambersburg PA
CBHW031505270326
41930CB00006B/252